Body & Beauty Secrets
of the Superbeauties

Body & Beauty

Secrets of the Superbeauties

by MADELINE de VRIES

and ERIC WEBER

with LUCRETIA ROBERTSON

Illustrations by Catherine Clayton Purnell

G. P. PUTNAM'S SONS   NEW YORK

The author gratefully acknowledges permission to quote from the following: Eugene O'Neill *Anna Christie* copyright © 1973 Eugene O'Neill. Reprinted by arrangement with Random House, Inc.

Printed in the United States of America

Designed by Bernard Schleifer

Acknowledgments

With a special thanks for all the friends who helped open all of the right doors.

Alice Cashman
Peter Chernin
Stephen Chrystie
Ro Diamond
Richard Grant

Harriet Greenfield
Valerie Jennings
Gene Kirkwood
Maureen & Eric Lasher
Pauline Trigère

*Dedicated to the eleven super women who
shared their beauty with us.*

Contents

Introduction

IT'S A SATURDAY morning in February. The phone rings in the hallway. Glen drops his crayon and reaches the phone by the fourth ring.

"Hello. Yup, I'll tell her." Without covering the mouthpiece, he yells through the open kitchen door in his squeaky six-year-old falsetto, "Hey, Mom! It's for you. Ann Somebody from California!"

Hmm. Who do we know in California named Ann? We draw a blank.

"Hello . . . "

"Madeline, it's Ann-Margret."

It's been nearly two weeks since that afternoon we spent in her sunny living room. Yet the voice is so recognizable she might have opened just as easily with "Guess who?"

"I hate to bother you on a Saturday . . . Is it an inconvenient time for you?"

Madeline smiles. Imagine! Ann-Margret politely asking if her call is an inconvenience!

"No, not at all! How nice to hear your voice!"

"Madeline, I've been meaning to call you for days but I've been *so* busy and I never seem to be near a phone at a good

11

time. I've thought of something very important for the book, and I didn't want you to finish without it. Cold water rinses!"

"Pardon me?"

"Cold water rinses! For your *hair*. If you rinse your hair with very cold water after a hot shampoo, it not only closes up your pores, it leaves your hair really *shining*! I think that's a terrific tip to pass along to everyone!"

Ann-Margret, in the middle of filming *Magic* and frantically busy, has looked up the number she had scrawled down and filed away somewhere, and telephoned New York at eight A.M. on a Saturday morning just to pass along a hot tip about a cold rinse.

"Thank you. Thank you so much for calling. And for the interview."

"Oh, you're so welcome, Madeline! It was fun. I really enjoyed meeting you and the book sounds terrific. I should be thanking *you* for including me. Good luck. Remember, if you need anything else from me, please call. I'd be happy to talk to you."

We sought out the superbeauties via agents, managers, lawyers, personal friends, in search of specific information. A shampoo. A mascara. A diet, an exercise, a cleansing routine. This was to be, we explained, a book of facts. Written for them, but basically *by* them. A way of sharing their expertise with women who, like us, are fascinated by them and their superlative good looks. How do they do it? What products and procedures help them enhance their natural beauty, and help them to stay that way longer?

Who knows what we expected to find? "Stars," perhaps? Aloofness? Temperament? An impenetrable, carefully manicured facade?

Were we surprised! They were warm. They were more than willing, they were enthusiastic! These gorgeous women with smiles that glisten from the newsstands, with the Camay skins and the perfect bodies, surrounded by glamour and buffered by agents and multi-million-dollar contracts, *welcomed* us! They opened their doors, threw open their closets, dumped out brushes and tubes and named all the names. Not one woman was disappointing. They are all truly and uniquely beautiful. In the flesh. In the daylight. Some, without any makeup. And, yes, they're all slender and fit. But the really memorable thing about them is their *specialness*. Their honesty and professionalism, their balanced and healthy ambition to excel. Their humanity. They've made the most of their physical attributes without losing touch with their inner selves. They are successful *people*, and it's immediately clear that not one of them got there on her looks alone.

We never—not for a minute—felt threatened or uncomfortable with their beauty. They wear it well. As Jackie Bisset said, "Being graceful about oneself is far more important than simply being beautiful."

They are brimming over with gracefulness.

What began, then, as a primer for makeup and exercise, developed into a book about eleven magnificent *women*. Surprising people sometimes, but always interesting and wonderfully human.

It may be hard to believe but nine of the eleven protested modestly that they were hardly beautiful and shouldn't be included at all. Five started out discussing their own makeup results and ended by complimenting ours. Diane Von Furstenberg praised our bone structure and prophesied that we would age attractively. Liv Ullmann admired our clothes and said she wished she could learn to dress as well. Suzanne Somers swears that there's nothing outstanding about her looks. She's just learned "to accentuate the positive and diminuate the negative and not mess with Mr. In-Between." In fact, she's so baffled by all the excitement, she said, that "I keep looking over my shoulder, wondering who it is they're all waiting to see."

And, of course, there is Ann-Margret on the telephone, Phyllis George kissing us goodbye, and Marisa Berenson marveling with us at the blueness of her baby's eyes.

I think that whatever we try to do as women—create homes, cook meals, raise children, fulfill ourselves professionally and emotionally—the point of it all in the end is to enhance our human relationships, to communicate with our friends and the people we love. How we look should never get in the way.

—JACQUELINE BISSET

We'd like to share with you all that these women so willingly shared with us. To communicate their concept of beauty as a total human experience, as an attitude, as a style of living in which their *whole* persons are reflected. It is a commitment to health. Fitness. Confidence and personal pride. Professional and personal accomplishment. Wholeness, plain and simple. The commitment to being the best you can possibly be.

We're inviting you to come along.

Sit back. Curl up. Kick off your shoes. Take a deep breath and forget the dishes, the kids, the office. You're riding with us in a rented sedan along a narrow road on your way to an appointment you've been trying to arrange for days. You're expected at one o'clock at the home of English-born beauty Jacqueline Bisset.

And you're late. . . .

Body & Beauty Secrets
of the Superbeauties

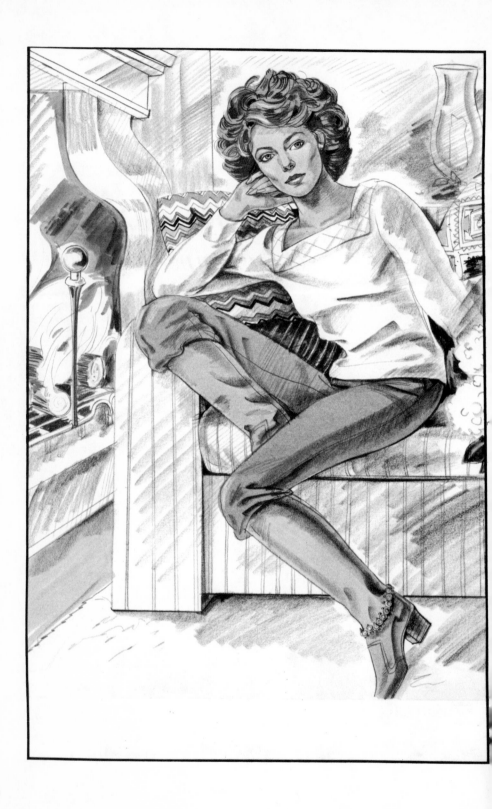

Jacqueline Bisset

IT's A WET FRIDAY in Los Angeles. We pull into a driveway off
Benedict Canyon Road, a few minutes late for what we have
been told must be a quick interview. The house is surrounded
by a high stockade fence; to the left we see a gate. No bell. No
intercom.

Do we just open the gate and walk in?

That's not as easy as it sounds. The gate won't budge. We're
standing there, getting wet in the light rain, taking turns trying to get the thing to swing open when, without any warning, an authoritative female voice from the other side says,
"Don't push. It opens out. I'll shove."

"Miss Bisset?"

"Damn thing sticks every time it rains."

She (whoever she is) throws her weight against the latch,
and there's a sharp sound of the gate bottom against the grav-
el as it swings open.

"There!"

And there she is. Jackie Bisset. Answering her own door. At
least we *think* it's she. We aren't really sure. It's not that this
isn't one terrific-looking woman standing here. It's just that
she doesn't look like Jackie. Or, at least, not the Jackie we

were expecting. For one thing, her hair's too short. And for another, she doesn't look—or act—like a movie star. Not at all like the hottest thing to come from England since the Rolling Stones.

But we haven't time to take a second look. Before we can introduce ourselves or make our apologies for being late, she's turned on her heels and is beating a noisy path across the cobblestone courtyard, her Frye boots clattering all the way. (Funny we didn't hear her *coming* to the gate. Could she have sneaked up on us while we fussed in exasperation? We swallow an amused smile at the thought of Jackie Bisset playing hide and seek with her two fumbling interviewers!) We're treated to a magnificent rear view of a pair of very expensive and well-cut suede trousers.

"Miss Bisset?" we venture again, but between the noise of her boots and the rate of her traveling, she doesn't hear.

This is ridiculous! You don't come to interview Jacqueline Bisset—Bisset of the wet T-shirt posters and the scuba tank; Bisset, the aristocratic star of *The Greek Tycoon*; Bisset, the Bombshell of the Bombe Framboise—and not even know for sure if you've just met her!

Forgive us. What you've got to understand is that Jackie Bisset isn't like any of the others. After having had doors opened for us all over New York and Los Angeles by a wide assortment of maids, valets, friends and lovers, we just weren't prepared for this. Never did we expect that the woman we had come to see would run out through the rain in a pair of suede pants, with no makeup, her hair tousled and damp, and shove open the "damn" gate.

The house is casual and cool and dark. She's leaning over the sofa offering it as a resting place for our wet things and we still can't be sure. It's embarrassing.

Then she stands up and turns to us. A slow, cool smile spreads across that expressive mouth of hers and we know. It's Jackie, alright.

"Well, hello, then! Awful, this rain. Come into the living room. I've a fire going there. You'll be more comfortable."

The accent should have been a dead giveaway. Even at the

gate. The confident accent of the well-bred British. So many people, seeing that name, have thought she was French. Many times we mention her name and are corrected. "It's Biss-ay, isn't it?" No. It's Bisset. Pronounce the T. Straight-out and no-nonsense. Just as it looks, and just like the lady. British. *Very* British.

We follow the leader again, through the dark, rambling Spanish-style house into a glass-ceilinged plant room with an amusing assortment of kitchen pots and pans spread around the floor.

"Mind the pots! I seem to have sprung a few leaks. They get fixed and then they pop again. I've about given up on them." She hopscotches around the mess and strides into the living room. It's an intimate room of modest size with a cool, grey flagstone floor and white stucco walls. The air in here has an earthy smell, as if the room were slightly underground. The beams across the ceiling and around the doorways add to the sensation that we've entered a cave. There's a fire burning in a small fireplace, built out from the wall in the style of the south of France. She invites us to sit wherever we choose and we settle into an overstuffed sofa, covered in rough white cotton and piled with brightly colored cushions. The mood of the room is very low-key, comfortable and casual. Not the least bit threatening. Understated. Just as Jackie is understated, dressed in soft neutral colors, her pale skin without makeup. This, we will soon learn, is the essence of her style. Quiet and unassuming. People-centered. And, most important, not at all threatening. She moves easily in this room.

She sits in the corner of another sofa, her legs curled up under her, her hands near her face. Her eyes are fixed on us as we begin the tape and the interview. Unforgettable eyes. They are cool, grey-blue—nearly colorless, penetrating. There can be no secrets. No hidden motives. No duplicity. Once she's caught you you're unable to look away. She can, if she chooses, play a little game of visual cat-and-mouse with you, lowering her eyes or covering them with her hands. But once you're hooked, you're riveted. We have the distinct impression that it is she who is interviewing us.

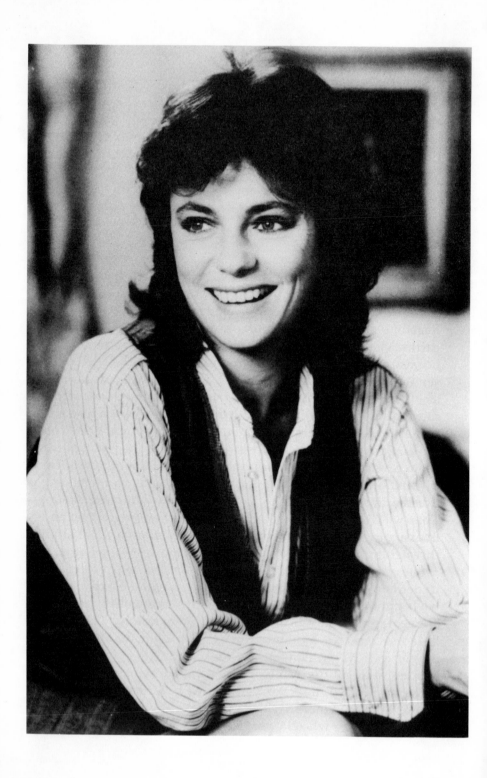

Her face, however, is a mirror, silvery and detached. Only her eyes register changes. Limpid barometers sensing fair and foul. She answers our questions easily and without hesitation, but we are aware of a certain impatience with the subject matter. Once she asks if we are sure anyone really cares about her choice of products or methods of application. Assured that a great number of people are very interested in everything about her, she smiles and shakes her head. It's an appealing, modest gesture. She describes at length her mascara ritual, then snaps us to attention with an abrupt "You know, I think most makeup claims are rubbish. Rubbish! It's all the same stuff, just put into different bottles with fancier names. You can buy it at Saks or the five-and-dime. It's all the same."

She may have something there! The effect of that statement was like an ice water plunge. Everybody stops. Then we all laugh.

Jackie speaks quickly and in a very low voice. At times we find it hard to follow, but after a while the style of her delivery—fast forward, pause, emphasis, fast forward—becomes a musical line and carries us along. We even find that we've begun to develop a slight accent. Her mannerisms are so appealing that they're contagious.

Somewhere, about forty-five minutes into the interview, things begin to change. Her hands stop their protective gesturing, leave her face and her hair, and settle into her lap. Then her body begins to unfold. Like a chrysalis stirring in a cocoon, she shakes herself out, stretches, and then rises from the corner of the sofa, crosses the room and plops onto a floor cushion in front of the fire.

Something wonderful is going on here!

The conversation begins to swing, to take a whole new direction. We finish up the fact questions. At this point, we invite more personal comments, more in-depth subject matter. Sometimes the woman we are interviewing has a little of her own philosophy to add, sometimes not. In every interview, this is a pivotal and interesting moment. We tentatively offer a subject: beauty and self-love. Jackie grabs the thought and runs away with the interview. Detachment and coolness vanish from her face. Her hypnotic eyes gleam and she drops her defenses like Salome's veils.

For the next two hours we share her thoughts; her appealing, breathtaking honesty about herself and her life. Her intellect. Her seemingly bottomless capacity for experience and enjoyment. Her reckless and nearly wanton love of living. Her complex narcissism, which has little to do with her physical appearance, but deals with self-love through the act of intensely loving others; a complicated process she must continually balance and rebalance to allow herself to remain truly free.

She is almost insolent in her casual disregard for her own intensely physical beauty. Her dismissal of her appeal is, in itself, wildly appealing and enormously sensual. She is never careless about herself. She's just beyond caring. She would never leave her house without mascara (but you are never aware of the mascara). Every touch, every trick, every effort, no matter how calculated, takes a back seat to her very centered sense of self and the electric strength of her ego. Something of this management of her own appeal communicates itself on the screen. In person, it is overwhelming.

"I don't believe in all those myths and rules about beauty. That sort of judgment is arbitrary and destructive. All it causes is insecurity. We really have to get past how we look and on to who we are.

"I don't consider myself in the least bit beautiful. I never have. So I'm at a great advantage in both my business and my life. I've never really lived off my looks. I can feel wonderfully attractive when I feel strong and healthy and loving, but, even then, the feeling is intensified by involvement with other people. I feel beautiful when I am making my friends and the people I love comfortable and happy—when I am drawing people out of themselves and helping them to relate positively to themselves and their lives. Being attractive can be a complete waste of time if it refers only to physical appeal, or to the prettiness of a certain dress. Isn't it better—far better—to have charm, to be pleasant, intelligent, able to relate to the people around you and communicate good feelings about yourself? To me, that's the real fulfillment. That's the truest beauty."

Jacqueline Bisset is much more woman than star. Whoever we expected to meet here, whatever glamour we anticipated, is long forgotten. The woman who came to the gate is so much more than that. Inherent in her nature is a set of simple truths. She is unflinchingly honest, in her view both of herself and of her role in the movie industry. She is aloof and she is fearless. She speaks her mind. Her needs and her goals are clear and up front in this city of hyperbole and hidden meanings. Here, in a business where reality and fantasy often blur into inconsequence, is a woman able to fashion a face to greet the faces she meets without ever losing touch with her own reality.

She says an incredible thing. We ask her what she does after waking to prepare herself to face the day. Her answer seems at the time to be amusing, but days later its significance stops us dead in our tracks. Here it is—the secret of survival for this gorgeous person in this tough business.

"I look in the mirror. What will I see there today? Who will look back and grin at me? If I'm feeling cheerful, *my* face is fine . . . just as is. A bit of mascara, a touch of this or that, and I'm off. But some days, the face that lives in my mirror just can't bear going out at all. So I create another. Perhaps this person will be better able to deal with today. I just paint on another personality. And then that personality goes about her business, a sort of Jackie for a day."

Those mutable grey-blue eyes are laughing. At whom? At the lady of one thousand faces who stretches out in front of her fire? Perhaps. Her sense of humor excludes no one, not even herself. We have all completely forgotten the time. The tape spins idly around the empty sprocket. Three and one-half hours have gone by. The first hour is safely recorded. The hour of facts and names and procedures. But after that? We're unconcerned. There will be little need for the tape on this one. No need to jog the memory to bring it all back into total recall. Who could ever forget her? Jackie Bisset is more than memorable. She is indelible.

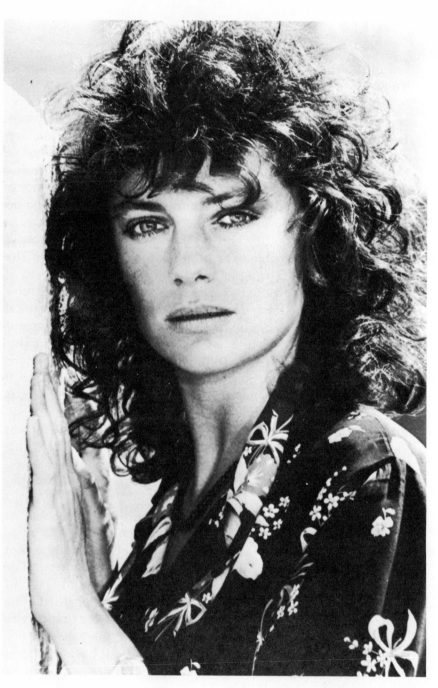

"I look in the mirror. What will I see there today? Who will look back and grin at me?"

MAKEUP:
Jacqueline Bisset

JACKIE HAS A beautifully balanced square face with clear English skin, mysterious blue-grey eyes set deeply under heavy brows and an expressive mouth. Hers is a strong, willful beauty, immeasurably heightened by her animated personality. Like her voice, her expressions are rapid and direct, and her pleasures and displeasures register instantly across her features. The overall effect rests on a basic principle: the whole is infinitely greater than the sum of its parts!

Jackie deals with her face as an entity unto itself, lets the visage in the mirror tell her how much makeup is required, and considers the most important factor the twinkle in the eye rather than a secret formula or skill. She's scientific in her approach, dividing her face into four parts and treating the angles she finds as areas of light and dark. She feels that most of us fail to be clinical about our faces and, as a result, get wrapped up in one or two features without ever seeing the overall picture. Disastrous, she says. The eyes come into the room without the woman, or the gal becomes all mouth. Jackie sculpts her facial color with two shades of foundation, sometimes to the complete exclusion of a cheek color. From time to time, she will use a dark foundation which hasn't a

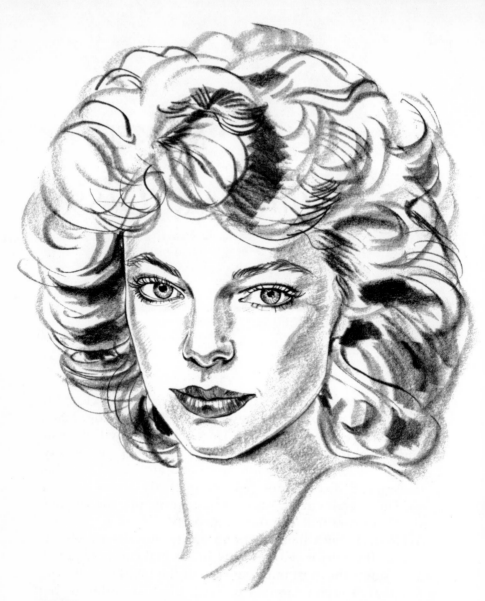

JACQUELINE BISSET

THE BASE: *Medium-tone, translucent pancake foundation. Sculpted lights and darks created with darker foundation. Brown or amber cheek color.*
THE EYES: *Deep brown shadows, heavy mascara, full dark brows.*
THE MOUTH: *Very soft color, Vaseline gloss.*
THE FINISHED LOOK: *Somewhat angular but healthy and radiant, glamorous but never glamorpuss.*

drop of pink, specifically made for black skins. Her favorite base products are professional pancakes in hard-to-find shades like "Chinese" and "Diabolique" which she applies with a damp natural sponge cut in a little square from a large sheet of sponge. This allows her a fresh, clean start every day without a trace of oil or residue to change the colors.

Jackie has a basic distrust of fancy products and feels that most cosmetics are similar—only the bottles and labels change from line to line. Her most prized cosmetic aids are surprisingly simple and affordable—Kyle Lotion, a body and facial moisturizer available at most drugstores; Lubriderm, another basic lubricating and protective moisturizer which she will blend right into her foundation when her skin feels dry; and that old standby, Vaseline, which she uses under her eyes at night and as a lip gloss by day.

Her lipstick collection confirms her back-to-basics approach. She owns two—a brownish-pink and a rose. With these two shades she mixes and blends "fifty different colors!" Her attitude toward lip color is, like the lady, very people-oriented. She rarely outlines her mouth or uses a great deal of color because she feels that makes her mouth "too aggressive." Nor does she use a heavy coat of gloss (to the perpetual annoyance of the cameramen!). "Too much gloss and I feel as if my mouth were coming through the door first. It gets between me and people."

Simplicity notwithstanding, you won't find Jackie at the checkout counter with a quart of milk and no mascara. The day can't begin until the lashes have been carefully curled and the Longcils Bonca, a French cake mascara that's a bit tricky to apply, carefully layered on, each lash gingerly separated from its neighbor with a straight pin and brushed again. She then flicks the mascara brush through her brows to even the color and shadows her deep-set eyes with a brown powder, applied with a Q-tip. She suggests that the eyelid be dusted with a little transparent face powder before eye color is applied just to blot up the natural oil that accumulates in the crease. The only time she uses colored shadow is when she is gloriously tan. Then she gets more exotic and dusts her eyelids with what she calls a "strange, dark green." The whole business comes off at night via Eye-Q's eye makeup removal pads.

Jackie's finished face is simply radiant—nothing artificial or "made-up"—including the light veil of transparent powder blotted with a wet sponge to remove the shine but leave the glow.

Diet

SHARPEN YOUR PENCILS. We've got a little math quiz for you.

Take 12,365. Now divide by eleven.

Answer?

1124.09.

Right.

What you've got here is the approximate caloric intake of each of our eleven subjects. Give or take a chocolate chip cookie. (Ann-Margret can throw the figure off a little, bless her sweet little heart!) Now that's not so bad if you realize that those 1124.09 calories are all consumed in one meal. Oh, you may say, that's a snap . . . a piece of cake! Now for the zinger. In most cases, that's it. One meal. Per woman. Per day. Seven days a week, 365 days a year.

Is this depressing you? But when you gaze at Jackie Bisset in a teddy on the rumpled bed of the chef who created Pigeon en Croûte for the Queen, you can see that the pain and the deprivation might be worth it. For some of us, the pigeon would be too much to resist. Not for Jackie. She has chosen the man over the bird. Self-love and self-respect over the croûte. She knows what is best for her and her health, and she does it.

It's a good bet that a vast percentage of the slightly less than sylphlike out there (just like us, we hasten to add) assume that a body like Jackie's is just naturally thinny-thin. After all, in her most recent film, there she is—laid out (literally) on a buffet table, surrounded by a seven-course meal. How could a normal, breathing person film *Someone Is Killing the Great Chefs of Europe* and not eat? And eat. And eat! She must have nibbled on the baguettes, at least tasted the bombe framboise, and we saw her swallow three mouthfuls of the spaghetti carbonara! Would you like to know what she *eats*? Really? Hard-boiled eggs. Lettuce. An occasional carrot. Want to know what she *loves*? Potatoes. Bread. Mayonnaise. Chocolate (and we could choke on this one) *icing*! But Jackie has her eating attitude totally under control. She's kicked the fat habit. Forever. For the lady whose most strenuous exercise is weeding, the answer was to re-educate. To eliminate the self-pity and with it the self-destruction. How? So she won't feel deprived, Jacqueline Bisset keeps (we shouldn't tell a soul) a Sara Lee Chocolate Cake in her refrigerator. As she passes through the kitchen on her way to work in the morning and feels the urge, she scoops out a big tablespoon of icing and lets it melt in her mouth for as long as she can. Just so she can say to herself, "Now that wasn't as good as you thought it would be, was it?" The "I can have it if I want it, but it's too blah for me" method of calorie control. Seems like a wonderful idea for all sugar freaks. A little indulgence now and then to keep from feeling miserable and being consumed (her word) by self-pity.

Jackie has another great idea. Her favorite pick-me-up is a blender concoction consisting of one cup of orange juice, one raw egg and some crushed ice. Froth it all together till it foams, and sip. We've tried it and report that it's delicious!

Like Jackie, Margaux Hemingway lives on one meal a day, or one small meal and a snack. "My whole life is a diet. Even when I cheat, I count calories. Yuk!" Margaux's lament. She lives on fish and vegetables—and vitamin pills, which she swallows by the handful with a bottled water chaser. Margaux, like so many of us, has never consulted a doctor about her vitamin supplements, but she did talk with a nutritionist in California who gave her a book and a cassette tape, which she listens to in her car. She swears by vitamin therapy as an antidote to fatigue and the blahs. Margaux does swing between extremes. When the moon is full, she may binge her way to bliss. Then, if she feels overstuffed, she fasts. Her longest fast lasted a full seven days. She described the fasting high poetically but cautioned that physical exertion must be kept to the barest minimum during fasts or serious trouble can result. In short, you can't clean the house, feed the kids, drive your husband to the train and play a round of golf while fasting without a rather dramatic finale. We suggest you consult your local physician.

Inspired by her mention of "binges," we asked Margaux about junk food and sweets. She replied that she never eats junk and that sitting in the lotus position was her only dessert.

Marisa Berenson is a vegetarian, not a dabbler, but a full-time, ten-year veteran. She's been known to while away the dinner hour sitting at her hostess's table, idly picking out the vegetables in the beef ragout and pushing the meat to the side of the Royal Doulton. Eating in this manner naturally controls Marisa's calorie intake. It's very hard to overindulge in steamed carrots and a lettuce salad.

Marisa's body is a temple of will-power. Looking at her lean figure convinces you that animal fat never passes her lips and that her spiritual sensitivities are never offended by eating any once-living creature. In this somewhat vague and dreamy girl lives one of the most appealing purists we've ever met. She never smokes, doesn't drink, eats no casual calories and the results are a testimony to her whole style of living rather than a simple diet. Marisa is not a flag-waver about her regimen. She simply and quietly picks the beets over the barbecue every time.

Not so Ann-Margret. If the richest thing on Marisa's cocktail table was the cymbidium orchid, the homemade chocolate chip cookies we passed back and forth in Ann-Margret's living room could have put a sugar addict into a hypoglycemic state. Ann-Margret is *mad* about sweets. She admitted to having tipped the scales at 134 two summers ago. (That's when she started jogging.) And when you talk with her face to face, this girl with the down-home sweetness and warmth, you can just see her sneaking a goody from the cookie jar, grinning in honest amusement at her lack of willpower. But in the entertainment business, when you appear on stage barely covered by sequins and feathers, self-indulgence is just not salable. And the firm and curvaceous A-M we interviewed didn't look at all like a nibbler. Though she loves to indulge her sweet tooth, Ann-Margret is the first to put a stop to her noshing when she starts to gain weight. She suggests the Ann-Margret grapefruit diet. Just grapefruit. And water. Punto. Period. For three long, growling, miserable days. It is, if perhaps a bit extreme, a real door-slammer on creeping weight gain. She does caution that you be in top physical condition before you try it or it can close the door on you for keeps. Best to be under a doctor's care. And never do it for more than three days. For a woman who passes breakfast by, drinks only Red Zinger and other exotic teas, has a quick sandwich for lunch and then (horrors!) goes all out at dinner, quick but dramatic little diets like this one have kept her weight under control without depriving her of the things she loves best. We'll say this much— those bite-size costumes she stores in her at-home wardrobe closet couldn't hide a figure problem. Whatever she's doing, it works!

Cheryl Ladd is another breakfast skipper. Seems that Cheryl is up at 5:30 every day. The only thing she can face at that ungodly hour is coffee. Black. In fact, coffee pushes her through hectic mornings on a caffeine high. She takes it "intravenously," as she puts it. At about one the entire cast breaks for lunch. Let us tell you about Cheryl's lunch. First of all, have you seen her lately? Hers is a body without a flaw. She's as delicate as a sparrow. Would you like to guess what this little bird consumed while we picked at our yogurt and fruit and sipped diet soda? A . . . cheeseburger. And . . . French fries. And (you called it!) . . . a Coke! You've got to love her for it. It's so all-American it fairly hums the "Star Spangled Banner." But her *binges* are far more international. She twinkles as she admits to a passion for chocolate mousse. And Beluga caviar. (Why, just last night she sat around nibbling until she finished an entire tin of caviar! Can you imagine?) And escargots. She *loves* escargots bourguignons. Cheryl's taste for wildly exotic foods is legend. She will make dinner of the hors d'oeuvres if they please her adventurous palate more than the main course. Says Ladd, "I guess it comes from growing up in South Dakota where the most exotic food we ever ate was French-fried shrimp. Dinner was always meat and potatoes, meat and potatoes . . . and then, for a big change, we'd have meat and rice. Give me a good chocolate mousse!" She's the classic kid in the candy shop! She also weighs a whopping 102. When she gets up to 105, she simply stops eating till she's back to 102 again. But, oh! Those three pounds! They read like the menu at Maxime's! And telling us about them, her eyes, barely visible over the sesame seed hamburger bun, just glisten!

Once upon a time, a pleasant-looking blond actress auditioned for a bit part in *Starsky and Hutch*. Her performance was good. She got the part. Then, a few hours later a call came from the producer. He was terribly sorry, but they had just seen the test, and she shot too heavy. She was too chunky for television.

The girl's name was Suzanne Somers.

Chrissy with a weight problem? Never, you say. Suzanne was one of those skinny kids who could eat anything and not gain an ounce. Then, suddenly, it all changed. Practically overnight, the pounds started sneaking on. Is this a familiar story? How many of us have experienced this sudden turnaround of metabolism during adolescence, or after the first or second baby? Who knows what sets it off? As Suzanne says, "One day I just started putting it on, I guess, a little at a time. I always thought of myself as a thin person. And then, whammo! Twenty pounds too heavy for the camera." The camera, of course, is brutal. That cold, mechanical eye automatically adds up to fifteen pounds as it slightly flattens out the body on the film. Did you know that most models and actresses are about fifteen pounds lighter than they look in stills or on film? It's usually a surprise to see them in the flesh. They're so *small* and *thin.* "That producer was right, and he did me a gigantic favor by telling it like it was. Then and there, I did something about it."

Suzanne found an expert, a nutritionist with a terrific track record, who helped put her in the shape she's in today. Need we say another word? How was this reshaping accomplished? First of all, the nutritionist gave S.S. a little black book into which she had to enter every single mouthful, every tidbit that passed her lips; every nut, every seed, every cough drop. The tally was astounding. There it was in black and white, all of those unnecessary calories. Next came the new regimen. Her new way of eating contained almost no fats at all. (Her top fat intake is three tablespoons a day.) If you think about this for a second, you'll realize that it eliminates a lot of foods and requires an entirely new method of cooking. Suzanne eats hardly any red meats at all; she sticks to fish and chicken, broiled or stir-fried in soy sauce. Soy sauce? Yup. S.S. claims that nothing can compare to boneless bits of chicken tossed in soy sauce over a hot flame in a wok, or chicken brushed with soy sauce, cooked until crackling under the broiler. Soy sauce has no calories and, more important for Suzanne, no fat. She says that cooking this way is addictive. Now she prefers broiling to any other cooking method and doesn't even miss gooey fatty meats. We tried it at home and found it very snappy and satisfying. Butter never makes it into Suzanne's fridge—only diet margarine. And even though she can still eat a favorite, peanut butter, she picks the natural variety that separates in the jar. Then she can pour off the oil and eat the butter dry. Where there's a will . . .

We wonder what that producer thinks of chubby Suzanne now.

While we're mentioning recipes and food tips, Olivia Newton-John has a great breakfast idea. Muesli. Never heard of it? The original muesli comes from Switzerland and the Bircher Clinic, a famous health and nutrition clinic that people with serious health problems go to for rest and a diet cure. At Bircher, the wake-up treat is muesli. We've made it for years and find it to be a superhealthy, superenergizing way to start the day. Here's how to make muesli at home:

½   cup Granola (preferably homemade) or raw oatmeal
1   apple, cored but with the skin on, grated
1   ripe banana, mashed with a fork
    juice of ¼ lemon, to keep the fruit from discoloring
      and to add zesty tartness
1   handful of raisins (optional)
1 or 2 tablespoons of raw wheatgerm (optional)
    yogurt
    handful of raw walnuts or other nuts, chopped, to
      sprinkle on the top

Mix the first six ingredients together in a bowl. Add yogurt to taste (approximately three heaping tablespoons) and sprinkle nuts on top. Eat immediately. It is delicious. Don't count the calories. Consider the benefits of the raw fruit and nuts and the natural yogurt and start your day with superenergy.

Mary Tyler Moore is a diabetic. This fact of her life has completely dominated her eating habits for the last twelve years. She is in no way incapacitated by her condition. In fact, she claims that her sensible diet and the medical controls diabetes has imposed on her life-style have actually improved her general health and well-being. Isn't that just like Mary? She turns a serious health problem into a challenge and, ultimately, a plus. Each morning Mary has an egg and a grapefruit or some other fresh fruit. Lunch is ground sirloin, cottage cheese, and tomato or a mixed green salad with a light dressing. She has a normal, but careful, dinner with her husband. And she has insulin every day. She is a diabetic who is in good control and as a result is as healthy as everybody else. Her whole attitude is one of sensible living. She takes a multiple vitamin every day, gets into bed by ten-thirty P.M. and sleeps, as her husband puts it, like a real "dumbbell" soundly and deeply until seven-thirty in the morning. Sure, sometimes she goes a little crazy, eats a few cookies, and she does smoke (although she would like to stop) and does have an evening drink. But, in general, there's an evenness to Mary Tyler Moore that is in all probability the single most important factor in her terrific stamina, good looks and good health.

Here's a very positive approach to the body beautiful and diet, suggested by Liv Ullmann, to whom eating with friends is a valued social activity. Being convivial over supper on a regular basis makes the notion of dieting a hard pill to swallow. So, Liv tries to combine fitness through dieting with fitness through exercise and the pleasure of feeling toned, firm and healthy. First, she says, feel good about your body. Run. Do yoga. Do something active you enjoy. Then saying no to the wrong foods is a natural and a pleasurable experience rather than a torturous one. First the self-esteem. Then the willpower will take care of itself. That really makes sense. And it's only too true that if you have a strenuous exercise you love—running, for instance—you learn early on that you can't do it well on a box of cookies. And a heavier-than-necessary meal doesn't give you energy. It just gives you the yuks.

As you can well imagine, everyone we interviewed had a lot to say about diet. Get any self-aware woman started on that subject and you'd better have an extra sixty-minute cassette tape in your pocket. But of them all, the funniest and most human was Phyllis George. Among these amazons of willpower and restraint, Phyl's dietary trials and tribulations sounded so much like our own that it made us laugh. She's full of gastronomical foibles. Picture, if you will, a bleak, overcast, bitterly cold New York afternoon. No exciting appointment to dispel the gloom. The prospect of a long evening at home. Maybe the laundry to be done. Or some unwashed dishes in the sink. We've all been there, no matter what town we call home. On an afternoon like that Phyllis George can put away an entire box of Oreos.

Or try this scenario. Walking briskly through an airport (or the subway, or the bus terminal). Temptation. The candy counter. Anyone looking? Quick! Grab a Butterfinger. Eat it on the run. Don't stop to count. Just oh, boy, am I hungry! This will give me energy. It's okay for today because today I'm so busy (or so tired or so hassled, or so fat, or so thin). And then, the guilt. The regrets. A pimple. A pound. It's reassuring to know that a gloriously pulled-together TV personality succumbs, from time to time, to a 265-calorie disaster in an orange and blue wrapper. Phyl *loves* Butterfingers. And Phyl loves Chinese. And French. And Italian. (She'd walk a mile for good pasta!) And oh, yes, beyond all else, cheesecake. She can rattle off the pluses and minuses of all the New York cheesecake sources. Under pressure, she can nibble her way through millions of hors d'oeuvres in record time. In fact, she claims to hold the world's indoor track record for canapés. She dreams about great ice cream and has her own top ten Baskin Robbins favorite flavors. How we sympathize! It's all so painfully familiar! How badly *we* want to be svelte and divine. How impossible it is to give up food. How do those others do it?

Phyllis, as you can well imagine by looking at her, has found some answers to the above. Open the door to her refrigerator. All you'll find are eggs and open cans of tuna fish. Maybe a head of lettuce. One way to fight the urge to eat is simply not to keep anything naughty around. Just carrots. And celery. Lots of hard-boiled eggs. Tab. Cold chicken (broiled). And yogurt (plain). And egg salad. (For Phyllis, *The Egg and I* has another meaning!) And, when all else fails, she fasts. Or, if lying around the house isn't in the cards, she semi-fasts and snacks on raw foods all day. In either case, she drinks gallons of water to help clean out her system.

Phyllis also has gone cold turkey at La Costa: 600 lousy little calories a day. Beautifully prepared, of course—but no matter what the magazines say, you just can't get a warm, full feeling on aesthetics and a sprig of parsley served in the nick of time between the fourth exercise class of the day and a dead faint. Ask her about it and she'll tell you how much Americans overeat. How we don't realize it until confronted with those paltry 600 calories; then we learn that one can get by easily on that much—without keeling over. Then she'll smile and admit that she cried for the first three days she was there!

In closing, we can safely say that the discipline is as thick as clotted cream and the will to survive temptation and stay thin is ironclad. There's no room for failure. These gals mean business. Each may have her own route to superslim, but they all agree on one diet control. Fall in love. It's hard to remember a roast beef sandwich in a clinch. Love can cause even the most weak-willed dieter to forget everything but the moment at hand. And if there isn't a man who can hold a candle to your mother's apple pie, follow the White Queen's advice to little Alice in Wonderland: "The rule is, jam tomorrow and jam yesterday—but never jam today."

Ann-Margret

A CALICO CAT is sunning himself on the walk. At the sound of
the car door he stretches, takes a long sloe-eyed look, blinks
and falls asleep. The air is fresh and soft and there's the sound
of insects humming in the field that separates the other buildings from the main house. We've heard that Humphrey Bogart
and Lauren Bacall lived here, years ago. Were they the ones
who named this hilltop estate "Hedgerow Farm"? You can
almost picture Bogie in his overalls and Betty Bacall in old
dungarees and a sunhat, planting flowers.

We head for the house, past the tractor shed with its resident vintage Rolls-Royce, across the pool terrace and up to the
front door. The door is white, bracketed by flower beds— as
unpretentious and "just folks" as a Norman Rockwell illustra-
tion for the *Saturday Evening Post*. Picture perfect.

Bogie and Bacall have long since gone from these bucolic
seven acres and the Hollywood farmhouse. The newest own-
ers are Roger Smith and his wife, Ann-Margret.

Richard Grant answers the door chime. It was Richard who
arranged for us to get past the huge iron gate at the foot of the
hill, past the cat and the snapdragons and into this picture-
book house. He's got such a friendly smile that it's hard to

39

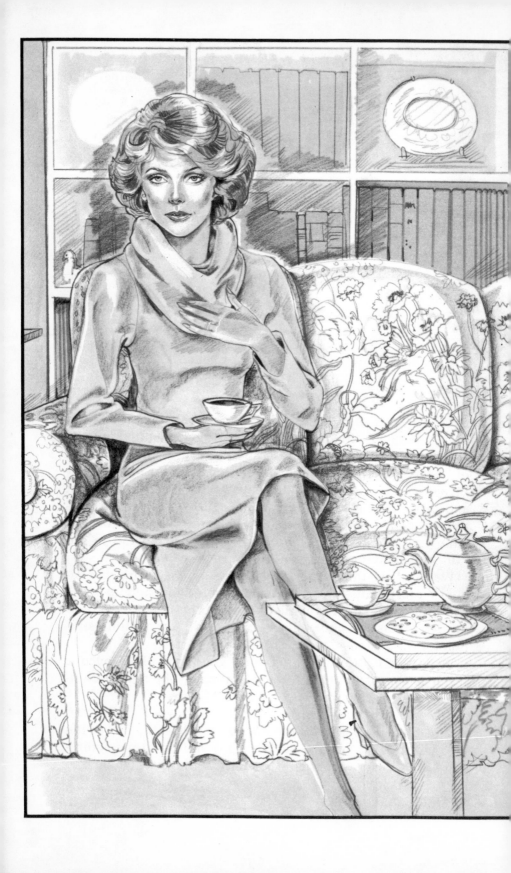

believe he's one of the most powerful and influential press agents in show business. We're welcomed like old friends. It's very nice. He leads us through the small foyer and into the living room.

If you were asked to describe, sight unseen, Ann-Margret's living room, what would come to mind? Flowers? Yes, bouquets of flowers. Floral chintzes on curvaceous sofas and side chairs. Roses, tulips, pansies . . . a profusion of blooms, covering everything from the toss pillows to the hand-painted, seven-foot room screen. And the colors? Pastels. Soft, but not timid. Cosmetic pinks, baby blues. Greens as zesty as spearmint candy. Everything lit by the sun and two crystal chandeliers, dangling like a pair of diamond earrings. A parade of confetti-colored paintings in bleached blond frames lining the walls. And a Steinway grand, resplendent in the bay window. The whole room is as profusely floral as expensive French perfume—a little sensual, a little heady—as if in anticipation of a romantic evening.

It's a *wonderful* room. Chock-full of things to look at. Intensely personal, carefully orchestrated, friendly. Sure, you might say, I couldn't live with those chandeliers. Yet the overall feeling in here is light, sunny and very pretty.

On a silent cue, Ann-Margret enters the room. (No Loretta Young entrance. She simply stands there and smiles.) We recognize her instantly! That famous strawberry blond hair. The soft, pouting mouth. The dancer's body—all legs. (She's shorter than we expected.)

We can't help ourselves. We're experiencing flashbacks. Pat Boone. Elvis. Carhops and convertibles and drive-in movies. All those flicks of the early Sixties whose names we've forgotten. And Ann-Margret, full of enviable and innocent sexuality, tossing her foot-long ponytail in time with the rock guitars. (Her hair is so *orderly*.) Ann-Margret and Elvis in *Viva Las Vegas!* Ann-Margret on a marquee in a flash of head-to-toe sequins. (Her dress is so modest—almost suburban!) She says good morning and there's that unmistakable purring voice, an instant replay of every inviting line she's ever delivered up there on the giant screen. (She offers us homemade chocolate chip cookies and tea.) We can hardly wait to ask her: tell us, what's it like, dressing up in laces and feathers and dancing for the camera—being a beauty queen—is it fun? (A little bit of chocolate sticks to the back of her finger. She good-naturedly swipes at it with the tip of her tongue and smiles at us.)

"A beauty? I never thought of myself as a beauty. Never in my life. Of course, there was a lot of studio publicity, but I never believed any of it. As a matter of fact, I was very flattered when Richard told me that you wanted to talk with me. It's funny, me in a beauty book. You know, when I was growing up, my parents' friends would say, isn't she a nice little girl, a polite little girl, or, isn't she talented? But no one ever called me beautiful, not even my own parents. I was raised in a strict Swedish home with lots of discipline and lots of love. One balancing the other. The important things were family, home, friends, morality—never physical beauty. (She laughs pleasantly, remembering.)

"I had these two front teeth that were really crooked. When I began to seriously entertain, I had them capped. But, to this day, when I look in the mirror, I still see myself as little Ann-Margret Olson with the straggly dark brown hair and those two crooked teeth!"

Little Ann-Margret Olson still is very much a part of her charm. When she smiles, you can almost see those two front teeth, and immediately you smile right along. She's so easy to relate to, so comfortable to be with, so friendly that we're beginning to feel like school chums chatting away in somebody's dormitory room while munching cookies and sipping tea.

"You mention my early films. Well, it took me a long time, but I'm finally at a point in my life and my career where I can look at myself and say, yes, Ann-Margret, you really can act! It took a lot of films I'd rather not remember and two Oscar nominations I'll never forget to bring me to where I am today. When I left Illinois seventeen years ago, people told me I'd never make it in Hollywood. That life would be too rough for me, so why didn't I just stay home. I had very little confidence about myself and my talent back then. Just this dream that I wanted to entertain, to connect with people and make them happy. The criticism, and the bad reviews, of some of my early films, never stopped that desire.

"When I first met Mike Nichols, he told me he had seen *Kitten with a Whip* and thought I was very good. And then, of course, I did *Carnal Knowledge* with him. People say that since that film, I've become 'serious' about my career. I've been very serious about my career from the very beginning, since I first sang with a band, since I stepped out onto the stage at the Sahara with George Burns and was 'discovered!'"

We asked her to tell us what it feels like to be a movie star and she told us about her life as a working actress. The answers all came down to one thing: hard work. She is open about her professional drive and modest about her physical beauty. As she talks, she crosses and uncrosses her long legs, carefully tucking her skirt about her so that the hem never rises above her knees. Photographed so frequently in her Vegas costumes, no bigger than a polka dot, Ann-Margret is every inch a lady in her parlor. The word that comes to mind is *demure.*

From time to time we catch ourselves searching her even, delicate features for some sign of the reconstruction that was necessary after her dramatic fall at Lake Tahoe in 1972. There is none. Her face is soft and vulnerable and kind—and flawless.

"It was September of '72 and I was performing in Lake Tahoe, making my entrance from a platform twenty-two feet in the air. I was up there one minute and then . . . I don't really know what happened. I remember the stage flying up to meet me, and then everything just stopped. I was unconscious for four days. When I awoke, there were all these tubes and everything, but I could see Roger sitting there beside the bed. Just as long as Roger is here, I thought, I'm going to be alright. I couldn't move. I couldn't talk. My jaw was wired together. The left side of my face was smashed in. Roger told me what had happened and where I was. He didn't try to convince me that I was fine. We both knew it would be a long time before I would be myself again. That there would be pain and a lot of hard work. But I knew I could make it. *We* knew. There was just too much to live for to give up.

"I might have carried that fear with me for the rest of my life, reliving the fall over and over again. But a strange thing happened. Right after I got home from the hospital, I found out that my father had cancer. He was in enough pain without worrying about my condition. He was so worried that I was crippled for life I had to prove to him that I was going to be alright. At least I could take that off his mind. The only way I could do that was to get back up on stage and perform again. So, ten weeks after the accident, I climbed back up and did the show for my father. The wonderful thing was that it helped us both. It gave us both a belief in ourselves and the strength to face whatever would come along next."

Ann-Margret is lovely, hardworking, modest and demure. And the spun-sugar lady with the silky voice and the Emerald City eyes has guts.

It's nearly time for us to leave. But in a spurt of camaraderie, she invites us on a quick tour of the house. It's not for a second that she wants to show it off. We don't feel we're supposed to be impressed. She seems to be having a good time and simply wants to share a few more minutes. So off we go! Her spirit is contagious. We're all part of a little adventure, going from room to room, getting to know her even better at each stop. First there's the master bedroom, all pink and white with its hand-painted furniture (flowers, of course) and king-sized canopy bed. ("It's got a water mattress," she confides with a grin. Now there's a significant combination, a white lacy canopy and a water bed!) We spend a long time browsing through her endless closets and dressing room with its make-up mirrors and retractable hair dryer. Her clothing is sorted and stored in special drawers and shelves, but last year's Christmas cards are piled in disorder in a corner. ("That's just like me," she laughs. "Every earring in its place but my whole life in a mess. I just never have time for anything.") Through the bath with its magnificent marble tub. We bypass the kitchen. ("Roger's cooking up something or other in there.") There are no children's rooms here, no nursery. ("A child is the one

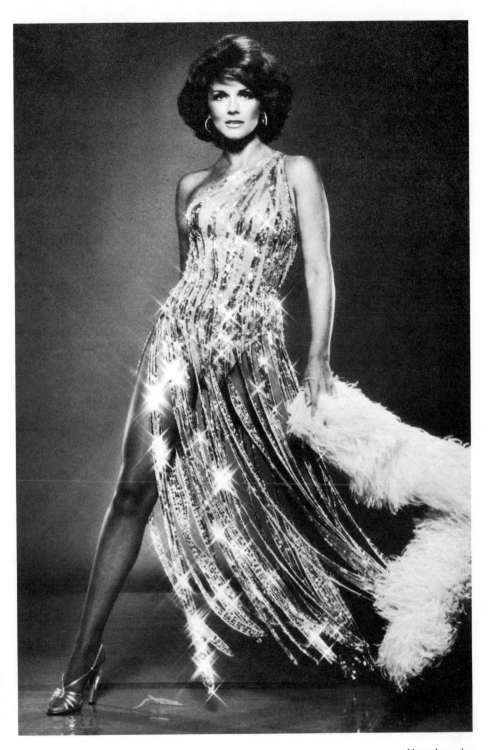

Harry Langdon

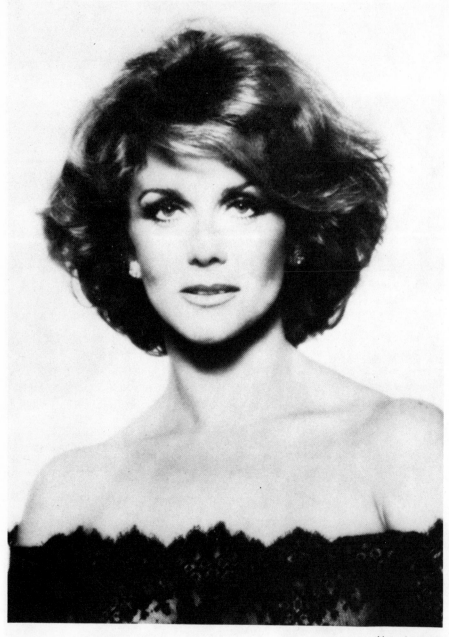

Harry Langdon

"But, to this day, when I look in the mirror, I still see myself as little Ann-Margret Olson with the straggly dark brown hair and those crooked teeth!"

thing I want most but so far . . ." Ann-Margaret forces a smile and shakes her head. The sadness in her voice is penetrating.) Then, hey! Downstairs, we find the game room. There, in the center of a plaid and dark paneled room, full of games and sound and video systems, is a pinball machine with a likeness of Ann-Margret. Shades of *Tommy* and the "Pinball Wizard." There's a small bar, and then down two more steps and into another large closet. But this one's different. This one is magic. It's stuffed from floor to ceiling with costumes.

Ann-Margret's whole face lights up as she yanks the glittering bits and pieces off the hangers and holds them up for us to see. She moves along the racks, pulling out the tips and corners of boas, breakaway gowns, tights. "This one was for . . ." and "I wore that on . . ." The upstairs closets were a wonder, full of cashmeres and silks and jerseys, but we understand now—watching her as she topples the hats down from the shelves and flips through the crinolines—that it is here where she is truly at home. Down here in this basement wonderland of paste diamonds as big as the Ritz. She is searching for the costume she wore the night she played the White House. They say it was the first time a Vegas show appeared on Pennsylvania Avenue. She was an enormous success, dancing in her red sequinned outfit and rubbing shoulders with politicians from Boston and the Bible Belt. Ann-Margret and the Gerald Fords. Knowing her as we feel we do now, we understand it all. The red-sequinned lady with the sweetness of the girl next door. She's having a ball. And we're loving her enjoyment. Clearly Ann-Margret is approaching the zenith of her professional life. She is the highest-paid female performer in Las Vegas, her television specials are always at the top of the Neilsens and she has evolved into a mature actress of enormous strength and power. But Little Ann-Margret Olson from Fox Lake, Illinois, with the lank brown hair and the two crooked teeth, is shining on us, here in this little basement room, like the star she is.

MAKEUP:
Ann-Margret

THE FIRST TIME Ann-Margret picked up a lipstick, she was seventeen years old. Today, seventeen years after leaving her childhood home, she owns hundreds. So many, in fact, that she opened a drawer the other day and discovered fifteen tubes she'd forgotten were there.

Ann-Margret has girl-next-door features and a little, heart-shaped face. But her years of practice and enthusiastic interest in makeup and makeup techniques allow her to turn that face into glamorous with a few flicks of the brush. It's all in knowing how, she says. She starts with the basics—the best cleansing and toning lotions and an under makeup base from France called Elastoseve Base from René Guinot which she buys at Aida Thibiant's Salon in Beverly Hills. Over this she applies brown contour cream in the hollows of her cheeks and, at her husband's suggestion, on the sides of her nose to sharpen its line. Sometimes she uses a little light base color, but more often than not she simply powders. The cheek colors are brushed on so that she can control them easily. To turn this powdery, soft look into a healthy gleam without shine, she sprays a mist of Evian mineral water over her entire face and lets it dry. The basic makeup is then set for the day. If she

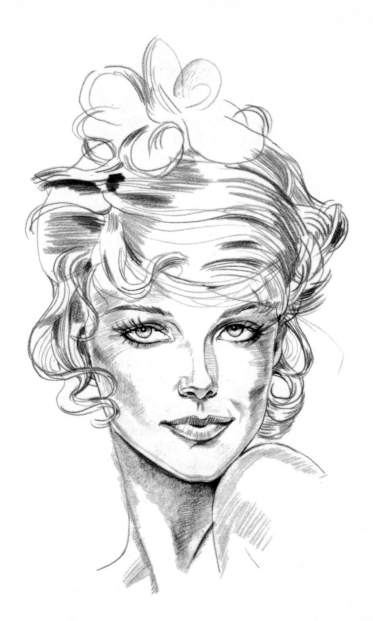

ANN-MARGRET

THE BASE: *Under makeup cream, very little foundation, shadows
contoured under cheekbones and around nose with brown cream to
square-off face. Pale powder blusher. A spray of mineral water to set.*
THE EYES: *Neutral shadows; pale highlights; thick, black mascara; natural
brows.*
THE MOUTH: *Pale, clear colors applied directly from the tube.*
THE FINISHED LOOK: *Fresh and pretty but with a lot of glamour!*

needs to freshen up for evening, she redusts with powder and sprays lightly again. The powder conceals the pores without heavy foundation creams and the spray adds a finishing glow. The results are very pretty.

What about all those lipsticks? Well, you won't find any dark reds or browns among them. Even though the fashion is to deeper shades, Ann-Margret refused to change. Paler colors suit her better and she's more interested in looking her best than being the first with the latest. She knows her own style and sticks with it.

Even on those days when her face goes au naturel (she allows it to breathe as often as possible) her eyes get the full routine. She says she would never be caught without her mascara. With all the mascaras to choose from, she prefers Maybelline, hands down. Thick and sultry Ultra Lash Black, in fact. On rare occasions she'll use Lancôme Black Mascara instead for ultimate lashes, but she finds it too strong to use on a day-to-day basis. Her shadows are usually neutral, browns in the crease and on the lid, vanillas on the brow bone. She brushes her naturally shaped brows, tweezing only the stragglers and leaving the brow line as it grows. When the delicate skin around her eyes is looking parched and drawn, Ann-Margret goes on a ten-day crash program with Orlane B21 treatment cream. She claims she's never found a better eye cream and swears it performs miracles when used religiously night after night for a week or more.

Before calling her makeup a fait accompli, she always perfumes. Perfume is one of the great loves of her life. She will sometimes change scents four times in the course of a one-hour-and-fifteen-minute performance. One of her favorite scents is a natural oil made from strawberries that leaves everyone in the first four rows drooling. "It's good enough to eat! Perfume heavily right after bathing or showering," she promises, "and the scent will stay with you all day, or all night, long." And she smiles a delicious, glossy apricot smile!

ℋair

CONFIDENTIALLY . . .

Jacqueline Bisset confesses that her whole mental attitude can suffer when her temperamental hair won't "do." In fact, she may not even leave the house. Mention "hair" to Jackie and she groans in exasperation.

Ann-Margret gladly pays the bill to Dr. Norman Orentreich, one of New York's most expensive and prestigious dermatologists, to revitalize her color-damaged strawberry blond hair.

After years of secrecy, a more secure Diane Von Furstenberg admits that her long, sexy hair is really naturally frizzy. Why now? Because now the frizz is in. "For the first time in my adult life I can take a shower and not worry about my hair. This is freedom. This is paradise!"

And Margaux Hemingway has perfected a technique for brushing her teeth in the shower, giving her conditioner time to condition in controlled humidity and without interruption.

Craziness? Maybe so. But in a nation obsessed with the notion of the "crowning glory"—spectacular, shining, come-hither hair—nothing is surprising. Americans spend more money on hair care and hair care products than the entire population of the USSR spends on automobiles. We cut, color, condition and crimp to the tune of billions of dollars in goods and services each year. Beauty salons proliferate like rabbits, hanging out shingles with catchy names. Hair We Are, Village Hair Hunters, Hairport, Shear Delight, and Welli's Twist and Curl Palace dot the streetscape in one suburban New Jersey community. Did it begin with *Hair*, that Broadway paean to freedom and sensuality? Or with *Shampoo* and Warren Beatty's swinging scissors? No matter what turned it around, the hair business has become an industry nearly as big as the national debt.

How important is great hair to great beauty? Very important. Perhaps more important than any other single element. Ask any man to describe his ideal woman and, liberation notwithstanding, nine times out of ten his dream girl will have long, gorgeous hair. Before all else. Good hair is more than simply sexy. Well-cared-for, healthy hair in a face-flattering, attention-getting style can cause an attractive woman to turn the corner to unforgettable.

Think of Chrissy. The image that comes to mind is that million-dollar head of golden hair. Not the ingenue face or the crooked little smile. The hair. Now, Suzanne Somers is not a raving beauty. (She'll be the first one to tell you that.) Charming, yes. Enormously appealing. But even if, feature for feature, her face ranks a middling score, her hair scores a big fat ten on the beauty scales. It has the sort of healthy dazzle that no amount of bottled blond can singlehandedly produce. But, to answer your next question, yes, Chrissy colors. Not a lot, you understand. Just enough to rev up her born blond for her character. The results are professional, silky and natural-looking, and have indisputably helped Suzanne become a legend in the Nielsen ratings. To keep her hair in A-one shape, she washes it every day and (super important) conditions after every shampoo; dryers, heat curlers and those killer klieg lights take their toll and a good cream conditioner helps restore the pH balance and the shine. Suzanne *never* shortcuts on professional care. Her word to the wise is—if you color, find a terrific professional colorist, the very best you can afford, and stick with him or her. Then all you need is a good cut.

Speaking of colorful hair, we heard a true-life hair horror story from Ann-Margret. A while back A-M performed the world's fastest quick-change with her hair color. She had been "using her own hair" (which, in show business, means working without wigs) for some time and it had been teased and blown and colored to near-exhaustion. Then she did a TV special and the producers wanted her hair toned down a few shades to a light brown. Fine. Abracadabra, light brown hair. Right in the middle of the taping she got word that one scene in a film she had just made as a blonde had to be reshot immediately. Presto! Back to blond. Now to finish the brunette TV special: back to brown. Shazam! Her hair shredded into split ends, broke off and started coming out in clumps. Emergency treatments were needed. Dermatologist Dr. Norman Orentreich supplied special products to start her horribly damaged hair back on the road to recovery. And drastic cutting was part of the prescription. When we interviewed her, Ann-Margret wore a simple, medium-length style, colored the familiar strawberry blond, and she looked terrific. All that trauma is just part of the game when you entertain for a living, she said.

"But I don't think I'll ever go back to long hair. It was always long, ever since I can remember. I cut it once at sixteen, and my father got so angry he didn't speak to me for two days. But I really believe that shorter is better for me now. After a certain age, long hair isn't pretty. It's aging."

Mary Tyler Moore has colored her hair for eight or nine years. That really surprised us. The object for Mary is to keep the original color, not for dramatic effect. She inherited a tendency to premature greying from her grandmother who, she says, was completely white by thirty-five. Mary's hair is a fine example of an expert colorist's skill. The color is perfectly natural, a gentle medium brown with soft, golden lights. And Mary is totally loyal to Joel Israel, her Los Angeles hairdresser, who has never made a major mistake with her cut or her color. Imagine the particular problem of a woman who has played the same character for years and is constantly filming new episodes. Mary's hair-length variations must be so slight as to be imperceptible to the TV viewer. In keeping with her even, professional attitude about herself, Mary has chosen to limit her hairstyle to these narrow perimeters. Her side-swept bangs (chosen to visually correct the slight imbalance of her features), medium length, medium brown, nonthreatening coiffure is as much a part of Mary Tyler Moore as her famous smile. And, like that smile, her hairstyle suits her well.

Most of the women we interviewed color their hair. Even fresh and natural Olivia Newton-John is blonder by choice. She sees her hairdresser once every three months for color, trim and a soft body perm. In between she, like the majority of women, goes it alone, armed with her trusty blower. Olivia has a theory about shampoos. She changes brands often, convinced that her hair builds up a tolerance for the chemical ingredients which distinguish one shampoo from the other, causing the shampoo to become less effective the more it's used. Interesting. We heard that theory more than once.

Phyllis George highlights her dark brown hair for very specific professional reasons. When seen through the TV camera, her rich dark hair used to look flat. Nothing lit it up enough. So she brought it to life chemically at Enrico Caruso's salon in New York. The effect was a new, softer Phyllis on the tube and a delighted Phyllis in the flesh.

"It was my biggest beauty change in five years. I just love it! I still commute for color and a cut!"

Phyllis has some very protective ideas about hair care. For example, she chooses to set her hair on rollers when she's at home instead of blowing it dry and heat-curling because she believes that's easier on her hair. She always uses paper on the ends to prevent splitting. If she must use the blower, she sprays first with Kindness from Clairol, and is sure to use a conditioner after her shampoo. She'll wash with Breck, but uses a special conditioner from Caruso. To Phyllis, the most important thing is that her hair be squeaky clean. When it's dirty, she feels plain rotten. She must be doing something right. Phyllis was named one of the ten best-coiffed women in the United States.

The most natural way to color/highlight your hair is with

henna. Nestlé was one of the original companies to sell henna in the United States and still puts out Egyptian henna in cans. Most health food stores carry some sort of henna and the newly popular "earth" products lines carry henna packs and rinses along with their musk offerings. As recently as several years ago most salons outside New York and Paris thought you were either a loony or a throwback if you requested henna. They figured that henna went out with Prohibition once commercially available chemical-based dyes were properly tested and deemed safe to use. The funny thing is that the old-fashioned grassy-scented henna mud pack is *still* the best thing you can put on your hair. First of all, it's totally natural. No artificial anything. Second, henna treatment coats each individual strand of hair and protects it against damage. Henna can work wonders, for example, right through pregnancy, when hair tends to break and become extremely delicate. In some salons you can choose your shade—red henna for fiery auburn; aubergine for a deep wine red; and, nearly everywhere, a colorless henna is available if you prefer the treatment benefits without the Flaming Mamie finish.

Both Diane Von Furstenberg and Marisa Berenson (front-runners in most things) have used henna for years. Diane began over ten years ago and goes every five weeks or so to Bruno Demetrio's Le Salon on 57th Street for henna and a trim. Bruno is a great exponent of the natural head of hair or its artificially cloned twin, the frizzy permanent wave. It was here that Diane came out of the closet with her natural curls. On Diane the look is wonderful and appealing, and much softer and more girlish than her Italian movie star waves. Diane's most important hair beauty advice is to buy a good brush and use it as often as possible. She may use a little diluted setting lotion for a more controlled look, but she never uses hair spray. With the frizzy natural look, maintenance consists, on the whole, of washing often. If Diane gets up in the morning to squashed or unruly frizz, she shampoos and blows dry. Every so often she will rub olive oil into the ends and then from the roots down the shaft to brighten up the shine. Result: hair liberation for the lady who used to hide her hair under a babushka when it rained and avoid vacations in humid climates.

Diane and Marisa have been close friends for years. And years ago they would take turns ironing each other's hair. Can you imagine the scene? Two dazzling young girls—one pre-princess, the other pre-movie star—doubled up over an ironing board. Was the setting for silk? We'll never know. Hair ironing has been phased out of the Sardinian folklore (the scene of these girlish escapades) and, like liberated Diane, Marisa has thrown away her iron and accepted her gorgeous natural curl. Marisa is known for her hair and the magical ways she can turn it into the perfect accessory. Wavy with this, curly for that, a chignon, a twist, or wantonly flying free—her hair is a natural vehicle for her expressive personality. Asked the secret of her beautiful tresses, Marisa just smiles and says that it's nothing, really. She washes it and lets it dry. The henna helps, but recently she's not using it much. Of course there's her vegetarianism which, she feels, may help keep it in good condition. Considering that a mere two and one-half months before, she had given birth to her little girl, her healthy hair was even more surprising. She did recommend Carita for natural herb and flower treatments, if you happen to be in Paris and have time for the works (Boulevard St. Germain).

We wish we could let you in on some well-guarded secret to Liv Ullmann's thick, leonine hair. She hasn't any. She just washes it and lets it dry. Somebody or other cuts it when she does shows. She never uses a conditioner and has no favorite hair care product. We might have guessed. Liv is very down to earth. There may be no secret treatments, but when Anna Christie comes on stage in the second act in her mackintosh, and the pink and amber lights hit her hair full on, it could take your breath away. Liv's hair is a natural wonder.

And, while we're on the subject, so is Cheryl Ladd's white-blond corona. Natural. Incredible! She has the kind of angel hair that makes the cover of Gerber baby food boxes. In fact, Cheryl's hair is so baby fine, she looked bald till she was three. But the final growth was well worth waiting for. Her hair is fluffy and, if not lush, well-nurtured and moderately full. She has never, she swears, colored. Not a drop of peroxide. So any "roots" you might suspect that you see on the tube are shadows, and that's that.

Cheryl has a lot to say on the subject of hair. She's very protective of her own which, because of her profession, is traumatized daily by hot lights, overstyling and the like. So she tries to wash it every other day rather than every day, and regularly uses a conditioning product called Extreme by Redken. She's got a habit of washing it at night, wrapping it in a towel and going to bed with it wet. In the morning, when she's rested and fresh, she tackles the problem, drying and setting with steam rollers. Even with all the fuss professional hair requires, Cheryl chooses to spend the extra personal time to create a little magic with her hair. She, more than any of the others, believes that hair is a crucial part of the overall effect and should be styled with your clothes in mind. For example, she will wear pigtails with jeans, a ponytail with fuller, softer silhouette, pull it up with combs or bijoux for evening— whatever the ensemble demands, Cheryl will do. Does it remind you of those teenage days spent in front of the mirror, experimenting with make-up and hairdos? There's something of the young girl, smiling at her reflection, that's really appealing about Cheryl.

"You could wear a terrific dress and have a strange hairdo, or one that's all wrong for you, and the whole thing just falls apart. Your dress might as well cost $2.98 instead of $298. With the right hair and a good sense of personal style, the $2.98 dress could be the hit of the evening! When you pull it together, pull it all together. Don't stop at your neck."

Cheryl doesn't believe in trendy hair. New is okay, but faddish is wrong unless it really suits you. Better find a few hairstyles that are right for you, your life-style and your features and use them as *accessories* to complement your total look. That makes good sense to us. Nothing too extreme or intimidating, nothing too contrived. Flattering and interesting. Just like Cheryl.

* * *

Then there's Jackie Bisset. The next time you look up and see her on the silver screen, tear yourself away from that incredible face and lush body for just a moment and check out the hair. In all probability, hours and hours have gone into that hair. Rollers and curling irons and goop and pins. And exasperation. And smile to yourself because you'll know something that no one else in the theater knows. Jackie Bisset hates her hair. It torments her. It causes her excruciating concern. It even affects her generally easygoing personality. And she can't leave it alone. She pats it, twists it, pushes it to and from her face as she talks. She despairs. She's nearly given up. Trouble is, the hair's too fine. It won't go, and if it does, it won't stay. Jackie's never had a hairdo that's made it through the evening. Somewhere midway, her hair goes flat. Succumbs to gravity. She always ends up in the ladies' room, tearing out the pins and throwing them all around as she pats and pushes and swears in total frustration. It's odd to realize that the impeccably together Lizzie Cassidy in *Greek Tycoon* was cursing the Greek humidity under her breath. Recently she thought she found the answer at a good Los Angeles salon. She had it cut shorter than she had worn it for years and suddenly she felt ten years younger and absolutely divine. Every hair in place. Bright, bouncy, she walked out of the salon a new person. Then she slept on it. R.I.P. The end of the hairdo. And the end of the foolish notion that this was a cut she could manage herself. But she refuses to resort to camping out in beauty parlors. She shampoos with Clay France, a product that helps add body and eliminates the need for conditioner. She uses heat curlers to puff up the top of her hair and add shape. Still, in the end it is Jackie's hair that's in the driver's seat. The condition of the stuff that grows out of that intelligent head of hers really molds her day-to-day self-image. If it's manageable, she manages. If it's good, she's terrific. And if it's horrid—well, she may just go back to bed. And that's that!

We came away with interesting information on the subject of hair. Everyone gave hair a lot of attention and knew a great deal about hair problems and how to correct them. Henna,

particularly colorless henna, seemed like a great idea. For that
and the olive oil we thank Diane. From Ann-Margret we got
the use of the cold water rinse and a firsthand warning against
overcoloring. From Olivia, the tip of switching shampoos.
Phyllis recommended using end papers and having the hair
highlighted by a good colorist for added zing. And everyone
agreed on the necessity of using the best professional help
you can afford for color, or permanent waving, but also learning an at-home routine you can handle easily on your own.
Somehow it's comforting to know that eleven of the world's
most beautiful and famous women are standing in front of the
bathroom mirror (even if it does wrap all around the room)
blowing their hair till their arms could fall off. Just like you
and me.

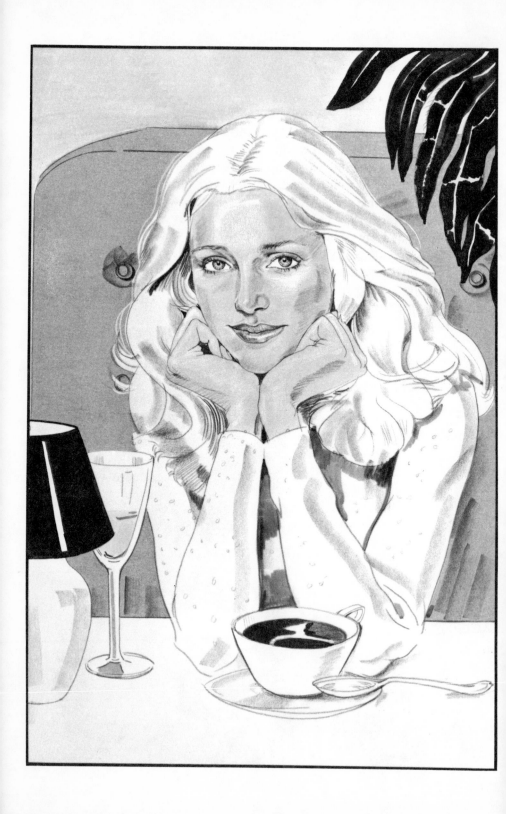

Suzanne Somers

"WELCOME TO THE POLO LOUNGE!"

Nino, the headwaiter, spins on his heels and plunges into the darkness, heading for the far side of the room. We follow, sidestepping the telephone cords that snake across the carpeting.

"I've put you at Table #10. It is a very good table. Watch your step, please!"

It's really hard to see anything in here but we catch a glimpse of #10, way back there in a corner behind a room-sized palm tree and lit by the purple glow of a plant light. We check out the faces at every table as we pass, looking for someone we recognize. The famous Polo Lounge in the Beverly Hills Hotel is the place to go, with a pen and an autograph book, any afternoon around five. Out in the lobby it's broad daylight. In here, the stars have come out.

Anything can happen. Contracts are signed over the guacamole. Fees are negotiated. The guy sitting in the booth next to yours might be packaging the sequel to *Gone with the Wind* or refereeing a professional reconciliation between Sonny and Cher. And all those plug-in telephones really mean business. It's a very exciting place.

But we're settling into Table #10 (it's a very little good table) for more than eavesdroping over the banquette. In ten minutes we will be joined by Suzanne Somers, the hottest property in Television City.

We order a Campari and a telephone (why not—they're free!) and jack in the tape deck. Ready, set . . .

> Star light, star bright,
> First star I see tonight . . .

(If you don't count Steve Lawrence who breezed through the lobby while one of us was tying a shoe. . . .)

Go!

In she walks. Now, you might think she could sneak up on us unnoticed in this jammed room. Wrong. *Everyone* notices. One after another, heads turn. There's a progressive lull in the chatter as, table by table, they catch sight of her or pick up the vibes. *Someone* is here. A new sound takes over. Dozens of people repeating a name like a mantra . . . "There's Suzanne Somers, Suzanne Somers . . . Somers . . . Somersssssssssss!"

It is The Entrance of the Star. Amazing! We never believed in any of that "star" stuff—at least, not until that afternoon. They're only people, after all, and she brushes her teeth every morning like the rest of us. Watching this girl part the crowd from one end of the room to the other with nothing but a smile, enlightens us. It really happens. There is *something special* about her. And when Suzanne Somers enters a room, she *really* enters a room!

We think about the speed with which this happened to her. One day "Suzanne, who?" The next . . . Suzanne is fond of saying, "Yup, that's me! Your basic ten-year overnight sensation!" But that's the only way to describe what happened when Chrissy was christened on ABC. Her appeal was stupendous and almost instantaneous. By the first morning after the pilot was aired, millions of people were on a first-name basis with her and had taken her up as the next *Blonde*. Suzanne is a network miracle. Yesterday a minor league poet, plugging her verse on local talk shows—today The Star, her crooked little-

girl grin lighting every newsstand with million-dollar sunshine.

She reaches our table and shakes hands. The busboys cluster
around her, pulling at her chair and gawking. Little Table #10
has become the center of attention. It's a funny feeling, having all those eyes riveted on you. *We* are getting the spill-over
glances and we find our hands patting our hair and straight-
ening our clothing in futile attempts to measure up. Have you
ever imagined what it must be like to have someone filming
you every minute of the day—public and private, and without
your consent? ("Ever since we moved into the new house in
Venice with all those windows, I've had this feeling
. . . well, just so they don't focus in on the more intimate
details, I guess. . . . We may have to move.") Suzanne is
glowing. We're beginning to squirm. Well, as it is written, on
with the show.

First of all, don't expect Chrissy when you interview Suzanne. Chrissy is the part she plays, not by any means the life
she leads. Yet you can't help but expect otherwise. Chrissy is
such a strong character. But there's nothing scatterbrained
about Suzanne. There are no dumb one-liners. The classic sex
appeal of the "dizzy blonde" is part of her, of course, but she's
perfectly comfortable leaving her TV personality at home.
Yes, she does remind you of other famous blondes, Carole
Lombard among them, but it's *Suzanne* all the way . . . not a
reincarnation of anyone or anything.

Suzanne is very much a girl of the Seventies. She's got her
hands on the wheel and her trip is under her close scrutiny
and close control. No excesses. Very down to earth about the
whole thing. In short, she thinks about her success, not just
enjoys it. She makes thoughtful, intelligent plans around it—
for now, and for much later.

The remarkable thing about her is that she is such a nice
person. Within the first ten minutes we know it wasn't necessary to meet Suzanne in this status bar. You could meet her at
a hot dog stand and have a great time. The potted palms and
the telephones and the $4.00 drinks don't impress her, and
she doesn't need to hide behind atmosphere or applause.

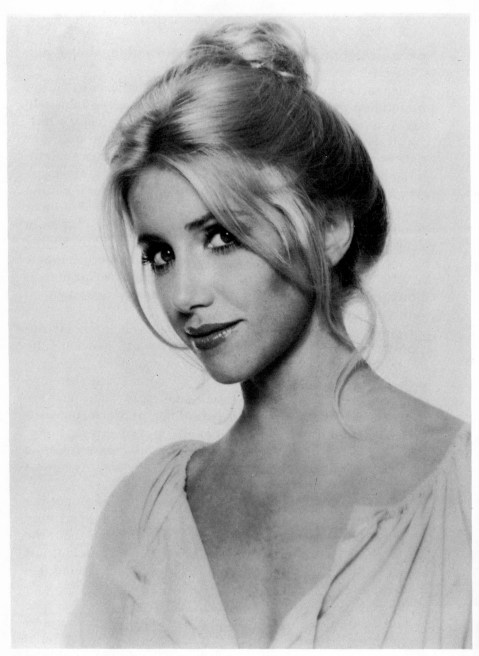

Harry Langdon

She's smiling at us, not the cameras, and she's enjoying everybody enjoying her. We're all—waiters and busboys and agent and interviewers and interviewee and assembled hundreds—having a terrific time!

What a combination she is. As we talk, huddled over the recorder, her comments are fantastic. Sometimes funny, sometimes profound. She's a sensational blend of good sense, good timing and good looks.

"I've been rich and I've been poor, and, believe me, rich is better.

"Let's get one thing straight. I am *not* beautiful. I've *never* been beautiful. What I do is maximize my good features and—this is the whole thing—have a positive attitude about myself. I look good because I feel good. Women who don't feel good about themselves will go to the grocery store with curlers in their hair because they're saying to themselves who cares, no one will look at *me* anyway. In all my relationships, I want to communicate above all that I like who I am on the inside, and I'm going to do the very best with what I have.

"Being pretty *is* easier. We're fooling ourselves if we don't accept that fact as one of life's great inequities. But no one ever said that life is fair. It's just something each of us has to come to terms with and then get on with living. It's true that there are fewer insecurities to wade through when you're born with a pretty face and body. But, in my opinion, the most crucial thing is not how you were born to look, but how you *feel* about yourself, your level of self-esteem. Often pretty girls can get by just being pretty. They never fully develop a sense of themselves as women. Beauty can be a handicap. Beautiful girls may never have to get out there in the real world and become real people. I'd rather be attractive from the *inside* out, wouldn't you?"

We'd rather look like her at this moment. She's one of the most appealing people we've ever met!

She readily admits to having early career struggles. Suzanne, the overnight sensation, didn't get there overnight. There was a quick marriage and a child who abruptly ended Suzanne's childhood at sixteen, then a divorce and night school and many lean years. But Suzanne never lost faith in herself, nor sight of her real goals which are not only success and fame but becoming a whole person.

"My real quest is to find the balance between my emotional and my intellectual abilities, to bring these two factions together to become a complete and harmonious person. I'm constantly working to synchronize my strengths in order to overcome my weaknesses, to understand before reacting, to communicate well with myself and with others. Professional success is peripheral to being a successful human being. Becoming 'whole' is a long and complex job. Maybe by the time I'm eighty, I'll have worked it out! God, I hope so. Because by the time I'm eighty I sure won't be making a living by running around in a towel!"

She wrinkles her nose and laughs.

The waiter brings another round. Thirty minutes into the tape and we're all gossiping about where to find the best sweaters for the best price in town. She pulls out her lipstick to check the color name. Someone makes a bad joke. We're all laughing and having a ball!

We like one another. It's impossible not to like her and she makes us feel like we're chums. What an afternoon! But the greatest part is that, with Suzanne, there's no such thing as a one-afternoon stand. Weeks later, she's having lunch in one of New York's chic eateries, Orsini's, when one of us walks in and is seated across the room from her. Minutes later, a napkin with a scribbled message is brought over by the waiter. This woman with the special something, who has every reason in the world to remain aloof, has written on a napkin: "Is it really you over there? It's me over here! Look up! Suzanne."

Clearly up is the right direction. She's sitting over there, glistening over her fettucini, working that magic on icy New York. Turning heads. Causing those same spontaneous whispers. Three thousand miles from L.A. where everybody knows her face, the Orsini's lunch crowd can't take its eyes off *that girl*. She's waving—come on over. Never mind that the whole room is watching. We're old friends and she's used to such attention. She lights up the whole place with that Golden Girl

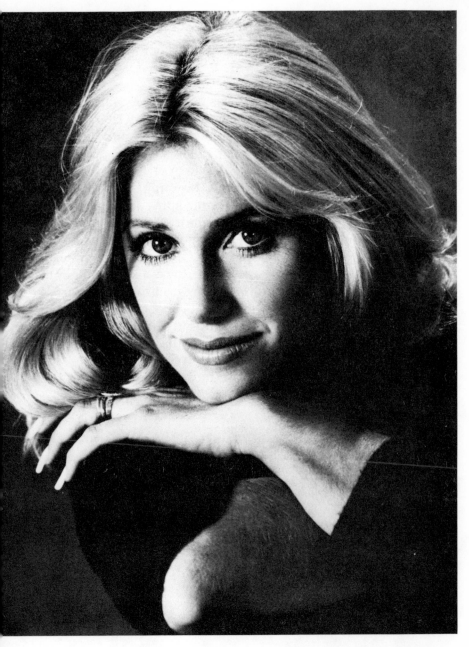

"Let's get one thing straight. I am not beautiful. I've never been beautiful. What I do is maximize my good features and . . . have a positive attitude about myself."

glow. They whisper, "Who *is* that girl?" Look up, New York! Here comes Chrissy!

One month after our Los Angeles visit, we are watching the live broadcast of the People's Choice Awards. There she is, shimmering in the spotlights in pink silk. They announce the winner of the best award the American viewing public can offer: Most Popular New Actress of the Year. Guess who? Of course! She walks up to the mike, beaming. And the tube comes alive. She accepts with the same spirit and enthusiasm that got her up there in the first place. The unpretentious, appealing girl with the million-dollar personality.

"I love to perform. Ever since I was a little girl, I've grabbed every chance to get up on stage. When I was a kid, I'd fight to get the lead in the school plays, which was usually the part of the Virgin Mary—I went to Catholic Schools. But my Daddy always embarrassed me. He'd sit in the front row for every performance and whisper to me, 'Suzanne, Sssssuzanne . . . get in the middle so I can see you. Get in the middle!'

"Well, Daddy, I'm right in the middle now . . . and life has never felt so beautiful!"

MAKEUP:
Suzanne Somers

A LONG, NARROW face sporting a big, broad grin, a glowing fresh complexion and gigantic baby blue eyes—herrrrrrre's Suzanne!

Suzanne confides she's just learning how to use makeup effectively (although she's been wearing it "far too long!"). Her resident experts these days are the artists who ready her for her sideline career as cover girl, and she's been getting into the dos and don'ts of shading and color contouring. To shorten and square off a lean and long face, Suzanne uses a nearly white highlighter to widen her jaw and sharply define her cheekbones. This creates two parallel horizontal lines of light across the face and widens it to nearly square. "Don't be afraid to use white," she says. "When properly applied and well blended, the effect is terrific." The blush goes on directly below the highlight (she uses a powder blush-on from Evelyn Marshall) to create her sunny, glowing, apple cheeks. Color concentrated on her cheeks tends to round out her entire face in a pleasant "glamour-girl-next-door" fashion.

The cream foundation colors are applied with a damp sponge so the lights and shadows blend perfectly. Even up very, very close, there's no shading line to give it all away.

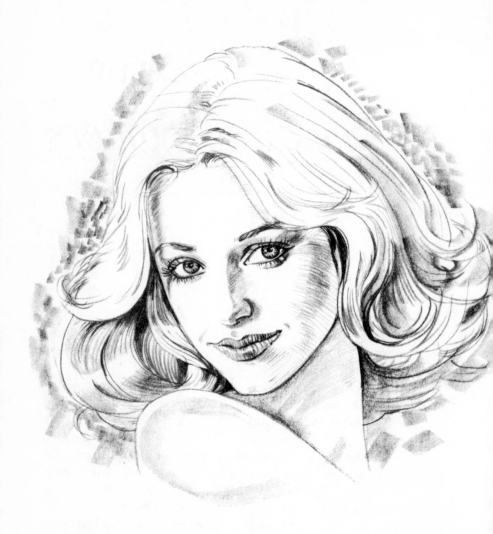

SUZANNE SOMERS

THE BASE: *Fair base foundation; highlights drawn across cheekbones, across jawline to square off face. Clear, rosy cheek blusher.*

THE EYES: *Medium brown shadow, extended all around eye; thick mascara; trimmed and penciled brows.*

THE MOUTH: *Outlined with neutral, lower lip filled in, clear lip gloss.*

THE FINISHED LOOK: *Face made more square, subtly altered but not artificial, very fresh but with high contrast.*

The powder blush-on goes on with a clean, natural bristle brush after the base colors have dried and set. Suzanne claims that with a little practice the entire routine takes five minutes!

And what about that famous smile? "I have a mouth that tends to run all over my face!" chuckles Suzanne. To correct this problem, she outlines her lips with a lip brush in a neutral color, and fills in only the bottom lip. Then she applies a clear, shiny coat of gloss over all.

Suzanne has wonderful, flashing clear eyes with huge pale blue irises. Her favorite makeup trick of all is done with a natural medium-brown eye shadow. Without stopping the color at the corners of the eyes, she runs the brown powder all the way around and then lightly down the sides of her nose. When smudged softly with her finger, this shadow technique creates very deep-set, glamorous eyes, *and* re-emphasizes the squareness of the cheekbones—a two-birds-with-one-stone gimmick that looks terrific. Suzanne used to have trouble with full and unruly eyebrows that, especially when photographed, were heavy for her delicate face. A makeup artist taught her to trim them short with a manicuring scissor, to brush them up, to pencil in the arch with a few light lines and . . . voilà! An open, ingenuous and youthful look that suits her to a T. She finishes her eyes with a flick of her favorite mascara, Maybelline Long Lash in Dark Brown or Black, and she's all set to meet the world.

Suzanne has learned how to maximize her basic good looks and camouflage her problem areas in some simple and down-to-earth ways that allow her to look her dazzling best without lingering long over the makeup table. And that narrow little face *is* a showstopper. Of course, her best secret is the one she shows off constantly—that happy Suzanne Somers smile.

Exercise

NINE OUT OF THE eleven women dance—two of them every day.
Five run. One jumps rope for thirteen minutes by the clock
every morning, six do yoga and three ride horses. Five belong
to organized exercise classes. One does leg lifts and tuschie
tucks in elevators. One plays baseball. And one swears that
love in the afternoon is the best bodily exercise. All eleven
can touch their toes with their knees straight.

It's enough to make you smash every mirror in the house.

The superbeauties really do look as good going as they do
coming. Not a one of them jiggles or rolls. There's not a dollop
of cellulitis or an ounce of flab. It's truly inspirational. And, in
nearly every case, it's a result of diligent, dedicated hard
work. Day to day taking care of business. Sure, a few of them
frequent the Golden Door and other ultra-elegant health and
fitness spas, and most have at least one organized exercise
activity for which they pay dearly. But what surprised us were
the number of simple exercise ideas you or I would manage
easily, and the serious athletic exercise these women do:
sports, dance, running and heavy working-out in a "man's"
gymnasium. As a matter of fact, it seems to us that among
women who make a business of being fit and toned, athletics

are rapidly replacing Elizabeth Arden and other such no-sweat salons. The switch to the tough stuff is almost a national phenomenon. These days, everybody runs. A pair of Adidas is as crucial to the well-organized wardrobe as a high-heeled pump.

Take Phyllis George, for example. When you look at Phyl, you believe that she runs. She is not, by any means, a thin woman. She is slender, beautifully proportioned, but there is definitely some USDA prime meat on her bones and all of it is toned and firm. Her legs in particular. When you see a photo of Phyllis is a warmup suit, the musculature of her legs rivals that of the professional athlete. Please don't misunderstand. There is nothing unfeminine about Phyllis' body. She's just taut. She glows with the flush of the marathon woman. But to hear her tell it, things weren't always so together. When Phyl took her first run, she collapsed after thirty feet. "It's taken a lot of time and effort to build it up," she admits, "but it's worth it! Now I can run several miles on sand (which is much harder) as well as on pavement, and I feel wonderful. In fact, the more I run, the better I feel."

Phyllis plays tennis daily on her private courts, as do many of the West Coast women we interviewed. This is, of course, an ideal situation compared to those of us forced to stand in endless lines for public facilities. But she also has wonderful little exercise tricks that don't cost a cent and require nothing more than a desire to pull together and get in shape.

FOR THE FACE:

To keep your facial muscles in tone, stick out your jaw as far as you can, then bring it up and over your upper teeth. (It's easier than it sounds. Do it in front of a mirror. It'll crack you up every time. You should look like a barracuda.) Now, gently, throw your head back . . . back. You should feel the tension and the stretch all across the lower portion of your face and through the neck.

FOR THE BUTTOCKS:

Next time you're walking down the street, work on that rear view! Gradually tighten the buttock muscles as you walk. Then, gradually relax. Do it as slowly as you can. Concentrate on walking tall as you do this exercise.

FOR THE LEGS:

Try leg lifts in the elevator! (We strongly recommend that you be alone in there for this.) Raise and lower your leg slowly. Change legs. If it's really a long, lonely ride, you can hook your heel on the rail (if one exists) and use it as a ballet bar for a mini-plié.

Knee bends are particularly effective on elevators since, one way or another, you're working against gravity. Be very careful with your knees, Phyllis warns. They are one of the most fragile parts of the body and can easily be seriously damaged. She's got that firsthand from the pro ball players. If you don't ride in elevators, try doing knee bends while brushing your teeth.

Try these two floor exercises at home: Cross-overs: Lie on your back. Raise both legs slightly off the floor. Open them to a small V and then cross left over right, back to V, right over left, back to V. Keep it up!

Nose to Knee: Lie on your back. Raise your right knee until it touches your nose. Slowly lower. Do again with your left, and continue, several times on each side.

FOR THE WAIST:

Just plain twisting is great for the waist. Keep your shoulders square and your hips perfectly stationary, arms at shoulder level, and swing with the arms as far around to each side as is comfortable. Then swing around a little more till it's not-so-comfortable! The secret to this and all exercises is to start with 3–5 repetitions and do just a bit more each day, ideally 3–5 more than you find easy. Easy doesn't count and it usually doesn't work.

FOR THE EGO:

Dress well for sports. Phyllis claims that she plays better tennis, posts better through the trot and schusses better on the slopes when she's dressed to kill. There's some good sense behind this. Certainly it's smart to invest in the best sports equipment and most suitable clothing you can afford. But, according to Phyl, the aesthetics of looking terrific on the court can sometimes make all the difference. It's a matter of confidence. And, even if you never get your serve in, at least you'll score a few compliments.

FOR ALL OF YOU:

Dance! Dance, dance, dance! If you can't afford the time or the cost of lessons, turn on the radio and let yourself go! Disco dancing in particular not only burns up calories, it can shape you in record time. Try working a few tried and true exercise moves into your routine. Stretch your arms high over your head . . . out to the front. Twist. Do a knee bend, drop to the floor, then jump up and arch your back. Head tall and stretch your neck. Perfect!
    Thanks, Phyllis!

If Phyllis sounds disciplined to you, you should hear Mary Tyler Moore on the subject of exercise. Mary says she has never not worked on her figure. Now, this is a lady who is well into her forties and long past the age when things begin to lose their tone. But to watch her move across a room is to believe in the power of determined mind over matter. Not a thing is out of line. As in all areas of her life, Mary is very professional about her body. She dances every day. We didn't know this, but Mary started as a dancer. She's been in training since the ripe old age of nine. She does other things, but she still finds dancing the best way to keep in shape and to keep her energy level high. Her idea of dancing is the real stuff: classical music and Margot Fonteyn. Dancing for Mary is an art form, not just an exercise, and it satisfies far more than a need to tense and stretch. To dance pleases her aesthetic sense. We could all learn something from this attitude. When exercise becomes an expression and creative outlet rather than a chore, it can be an intensely meaningful part of our day-to-day lives. For Mary, such commitment and physical pride are what fitness is all about.

Here's another inspirational story. Picture Marisa Berenson standing in first position at the ballet bar, practicing pliés with her chin high, her derrière tucked and her eight-months-pregnant tummy out to there! Marisa danced every day until she gave birth. She smiled with mischievous delight as she recalled how difficult it was for the doctors to make the incision for her Caesarean delivery because her stomach muscles were so tight and firm. Four weeks and one baby girl later, Marisa was back on her toes. For those of us who can barely squeeze into potato-sack couture for months after giving birth, the sight of a size-eight Marisa, lean of waist and firm of thigh, holding a ten week-old infant, was devastating! And inspirational.

Anyone who has blamed pregnancy for the permanent redistribution of all bodily assets should listen to Cheryl Ladd's story. It's uplifting, to say the least. Way back when in Huron, South Dakota, Cheryl was a cheerleader (can't you just see her with her pompons?) and a super gymnast. Because of the very specific nature of gymnastics (as is the case with many sports), her adolescent body developed along very strange lines. As husband David describes it, "Cheryl was Sophia Loren from the waist up, and Mickey Rooney from the waist down!" Actually, Cheryl had no waist at all. Her upper half, chest and torso, was superdeveloped. And, due to her slender, small frame, she had no hips to balance below. Now here's the clincher. Cheryl says that having her baby, Jordan Elizabeth, now age three, was what got her into the shape she's in. Jordan gave her hips. Isn't it a relief to know that someone has found "baby hips" a positive experience? Cheryl sums it up, "Since my baby, I've got it all together. My head, my heart and my body!"

Walk into any poster parlor in America and there among the alphabetized bosoms and bottoms, immortalized in a black bathing suit and filed under "T" (for *Three's Company*) or, more likely, plastered on the wall, is Suzanne Somers, television's number one body. Girl most likely to be caught in a towel. Prepackaged in a mailing tube and all yours for a buck ninety-nine. A gentleman viewer wrote to a national "insider" newspaper recently and claimed to tune in to the show each week *just* for the opening footage, or, more specifically, *just* for the shot of Chrissy in her black maillot. Then he tunes out. And turns on. Strange! But in the world of specialized girl-watchers, we're sure he's not alone. Chrissy's figure is a new national pastime. Now, if you're expecting that we're about to tell you it ain't much in the flesh, you're wrong. It's a lot more than much. It's enough to stop traffic. What we are about to tell you is that Suzanne hates to exercise. Can you picture those little teaser shots of S.S. frolicking on the beach and pedaling madly on her bike? Well, that's as much exercising as she cares to get. That and showing off that gorgeous bod at the pool. That's it, folks! But she's an over-thirty realist. Nothing is going to skip to the south on Suzanne for a long, long time. Even though she hates it, she exercises daily. (Toe-touches and situps, that is!)

If we were all being honest, how many of us could claim to love to exercise? Getting up in the morning to exercise can be torture. (And who can even *think* about it at night?) Staying in shape is an ongoing battle for Ann-Margret too. She works so hard at Ron Fletcher's in L.A. that it gets embarrassing. Seems she perspires so heavily during those dance workouts, she slides around on the floor. No matter. She mops her brow and dances. A-M loves to dance. And to ski. And she's a runner, even at Tahoe, where the air's so thin it nearly kills her to jog. What does she do if it rains? Simple. She jumps rope for thirteen minutes. She times herself with an egg timer so she never cheats. Sounds easy, you say? Try it, just once. Jumping for thirteen minutes requires the stamina of Muhammad Ali. Ann-Margret has had more than her share of physical comebacks and, therefore, understands better than most of us how quickly muscles can deteriorate. After her fall at Tahoe she spent eleven days on her back in the hospital. When she was finally discharged she weighed 106. (Her top weight is 134, so you can see how dramatic the loss was.) Her muscle tone was gone. It took her months to get it back. But she's a great believer in the restorative powers of exercise on both the body and the soul. Ann-Margret claims she can get into trouble, physical and/or emotional, when she just sits there. So she gets up. And dances. Or jogs. Or skis her way back to health. Just get up and get going and the rest will take care of itself.

Feline Liv Ullmann with her tawny, leonine mane and soft, purring manner and Diane Von Furstenberg with her dark cat's eyes both said that stretching was the only exercise they enjoy. Can you picture them, curled up in front of a fire, slowly extending each limb and drawing it back in languid delight? Of course, the fact that Liv came to our interview fresh from a baseball game could readily destroy that cozy image!

When we talk about exercise, we think of Margaux because, along with being a superbeauty, Hemingway is a super jock. We've got six full pages of single-spaced typewritten transcription of Margaux on the subject of exercise. The girl's a dynamo. She's also, of course, straight from the American wildly physical West where heavy-duty body work is the norm. She skis. She rides. She plays killer tennis. She jogs. She runs. She bikes in the park. She's a whiz water skier (she's best, she says, when there are sharks in the water!). She slaloms and she swims. Boy, does she swim. A little morning waker-upper for Margaux is fifty laps before work. And all of the above are just the sporty, unstructured activities in her schedule. On top of them, she does "real" exercise. She works out on machines and on a little rope gismo she attaches to the doorknob. Then she does fifty leg lifts. And a zillion situps. All of this totals a mere thirty minutes before bedtime. And what does Maid Margaux the Lionhearted do when she's got a few free minutes to rest and relax? Eat a bonbon by the fire? No. She walks. Just little walks. Like from 88th and the River down to the Plaza at 59th and Fifth. We get fatigued just writing about it. But then, she's only twenty-one. Things were a lot easier then.

The bottom line on exercise seems to be that muscles are in. Muscles on women are sexy. The well-toned and superflexed thigh has replaced the Betty Grable curve and the Twiggy sinewy stick. Being fit and strong and honed to the barest essentials is sexy because fitness guarantees stamina. And stamina makes all the difference in the physical sports—including marathon loving. Nearly every woman we interviewed implied that taking a lover inspired an overall upswing in muscle tone (not to mention mental attitude!). Who was the one who came right out with it, her belief in dallying her way to fitness? Unfortunately, we were sworn to secrecy. But we'll tell you this much. Finish reading the book. We'll bet you can figure it out.

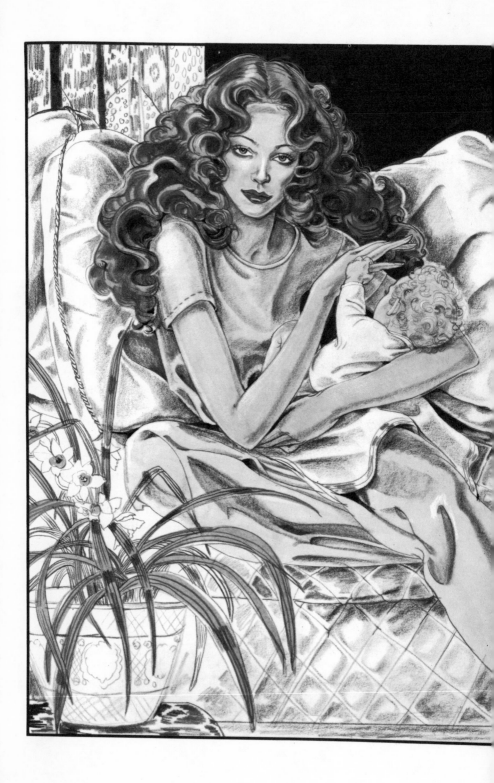

Marisa Berenson

IT WAS LATE SUMMER of 1968 when we met her for the first time. She was twenty-one and the top girl on the Ford Model Agency headsheet, booking at $100 an hour and out of the country so often we practically had to arrange shootings around plane flights to get her at all. The telephone bookers at Ford protected her every minute—weighing and balancing her commitments like so much gold bullion—to avoid overexposure. And once you *did* get her, the cost of a single photograph could easily escalate to thousands of dollars. But no one was counting.

The Revolution was all around us. Antonioni's *Blow-Up* glamorized the fashion photographer and his libidinous models. An entire theater company disrobed on Broadway and sang about youth and freedom in *Hair*. It was the time of the Beatles and the Stones and acid rock. High-voltage music, turned-on culture and drop-dead style. Out the window went the cookie-cutter dresses and the stiff, sprayed coiffures. In came the peasants, the gypsies, disheveled heroines with windblown hair and explicit sensuality. Out went the paper doll mannequins, and in came Marisa. The fashion industry had found the personification of the fantastic Sixties in that one incredible face.

Who could measure the appeal of that exotic flower child? Marisa reached all of us. She was the perfect alloy of good breeding and wanton sensuality. Not even the still camera could tie her down. Marisa floated across editorial sections in fan-tossed chiffons, suspended in midflight by Richard Avedon or David Bailey. Marisa of the luminescent skin, the almond eyes painted in dayglo color or ringed with kohl. Marisa of the perfect body, slender, but totally without angles. She was the vehicle for the new fantasy clothes and her body carried successfully what few others dared to wear. In the late Sixties, Marisa and fashion were an art form.

More than just another pretty face, this was a face with a name. Marisa was the granddaughter of that famous grande dame of haute couture, Mme. Schiaparelli; and, on the other side of the family, of the great art historian/critic/collector, Bernard Berenson. She was the product of European boarding schools and the rootless international rich. You could hear it all in that funny little accent of hers.

Before Marisa, garments had been identified by designer or manufacturer or, more simply, in print ads as "Left:" or "Right:". Now the reading public was offered the face *and* the name.

MARISA BERENSON in mauve chiffon from Giorgio Sant' Angelo, available in late April at Saks Fifth Avenue.

The model as superstar was born.

If Marisa was the personality of the times, more importantly, she was A Personality. Nothing she put on her body was more memorable than the girl herself. Anyone fortunate enough to work with her sensed that this strange, lithe fantasy creature who sang softly to herself as she danced and spun and created for the still camera was destined for a far broader audience. She was, in short, made in heaven for the movies.

When it all happened several years later with *Death in Venice* and *Cabaret*, no one was surprised by the lingering close-ups and profile shots, the lack of dialogue and the endless parade of gorgeous costumes. Marisa never really needed to speak to

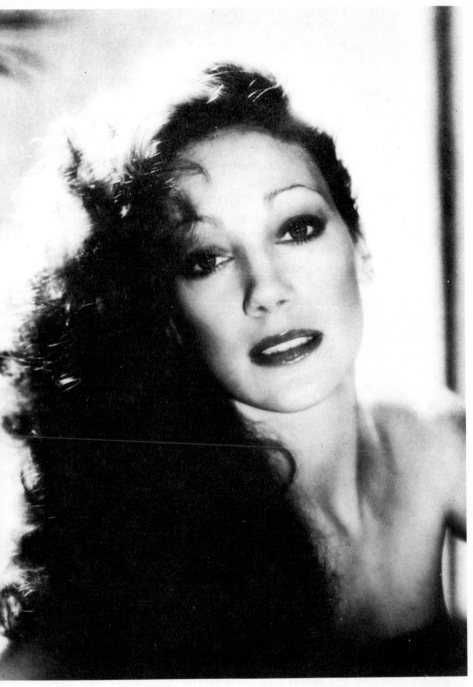

John Engstead

get her message across. It was enough to see her there, beautifully clothed and settled on a pillow. Having once seen it, who could ever forget the shot of Marisa arranged in a flat-bottomed boat in *Barry Lyndon*, her hair in a turmoil of ringlets, her pale, tragic face a study of loneliness and neglect. As an actress, she never needed Stella Adler. All she required was a camera and a good couturier.

I recall a vision of Marisa during the summer of '68. She was modeling winter coats and suits for publicity stills on Lincoln Center Plaza and the only available changing space was a dingy room in a transient hotel across the street. Between shots we entered the room unexpectedly and came upon her, standing by the open window, totally nude except for the thin gold chain she wore around her waist. The sheer curtain billowed around her, and the hazy morning light turned the contours of her white flesh into soft focus. She rocked slowly from side to side, staring into a large mirror on the wall, mesmerized by her own reflection. Perhaps she didn't hear us enter the room. Perhaps for her we didn't exist at all. She stood transfixed, her eyes locked to the eyes of the woman in the mirror. Not a hint of vanity or narcissism. Just a penetrating curiosity and an almost mystical visual communion. She was so breathtakingly beautiful that the memory of that hot July morning comes flooding back at the mention of her name.

Today, over ten years later, we will meet her again just off Sunset Boulevard in Beverly Hills. Our curiosity is overwhelming. Just who will we find there? The same enchanted girl grown older, or a businesswoman, parlaying her looks into cinematic fame and fortune? We're rooting for the former.

We turn onto the street. The house is a massive, freshly painted red stucco house, set up on a hill and fronted by a circular drive in which a gleaming black Rolls is parked. We pull up behind, park and walk to the house.

Look at that! There at the front of the building is what, for all the world, resembles a moat! A tangle of exotic plants grows up from the water and little islands of topsoil. We hopscotch across the stepping stones and up to the huge black lacquer double doors and ring the bell.

A houseboy answers. Yes, we are expected. Would we kindly wait in the living room?

Imagine, if you will, Scheherazade.

The room is a stage set for the Arabian Nights. A thousand and one objects to enchant the eye and delight the touch. It's a sensual masterpiece of flowing trees and potpourri in clay pots and crystal cachepots, plump satin pillows, overstuffed chaises, and color—color everywhere! Silvery lilacs, bois de rose, vermillion and teal, mysterious forest greens and the famous Schiaparelli pink. There's not a timid shade to be seen. Thrown together in wild profusion, this carefully orchestrated mélange of visual effects is repeated again and again in an endless expanse of mirrors. We are speechless. This is spectacular. Right down to the completely mirrored concert grand piano! The house is, to say the very least, the sort of place you either instantly love, or instantly hate. We love it! Instantly.

But just how do you sit in a room like this? Which of the precisely arranged pillows do you disturb? We wonder, does a satin settee wrinkle?

"Marisa will join you in a minute. Please, make yourselves comfortable. You may sit over there."

The houseboy has sensed our confusion and points in the direction of the banquette, a quilted lavender satin sofa that stretches wall-to-wall along the far side of the room. We thread our way across the marble floor, the kilim rugs, around tables piled with tiny breakable objects to our assigned seats. As we sit down, we nearly disappear into the overstuffed cushions.

What person could live here and not be swallowed up by all this hyperbole? We are totally unable to concentrate. Our eyes dart from one corner to the next, trying to take it all in, unscramble it and sort it out before she arrives. We must, in all politeness, focus on her person rather than her dazzling surroundings.

At that moment, a silent young woman walks into the room. She is dressed in screaming green. Fiorucci jeans, pencil-thin,

John Engstea

and a skimpy T-shirt. On her feet are fire-engine-red patent oxfords. And stretched across her lean body like a banner is a tiny child. It is Marisa.

Seeing her now, after all those years, we instantly recognize that special quality that kept the memories so real and so appealing for so long. She is unchanged. Not a minute older. The face is unlined, soft and shining, and without a trace of makeup. A mere two and a half months after the birth of her blue-eyed, blond girl child by Caesarean section, that unforgettable body is as lean and toned as the day she was photographed lying naked in the surf for *Vogue*.

As she greets us and settles into the cushions on the banquette, we notice that there has been a perceptible change in the room since her arrival. It is as if Marisa herself has given order to the chaos. It is she who makes the whole thing make sense. This house is, like the lady who lives here, complex and amusing, dramatic and terribly chic—a perfectly styled backdrop for Marisa who, like Scheherazade, is a spinner of fairy tales and has been known to turn a shapeless pile of silk scarves into a dancing dress in the wink of an eye.

She named her baby Starlight.

We ask her if motherhood has dramatically changed her life. She smiles politely at the understatement, and begins to talk. The voice is the same, dreamlike and appealing. "My entire sense of my femininity has changed since she was born. I feel the need to be rooted. Everything that I once accepted as integral and natural to my style of living has changed or is being challenged by this dependent little person."

The baby whimpers. Marisa settles herself deeper into the sofa and gently shifts the child into a more comfortable position. It is a gesture of awkward but loving tenderness. She is any mother, holding her firstborn, slightly unsure of herself. It is a charming picture.

"I wanted so badly to nurse her myself. But there wasn't enough milk. I suppose it's for the best. You see, I still have an intense drive to work. I know that I will have to go back soon, but I feel that I'll bring something new and more depthful with me. Starlight has opened up an entire new dimension to

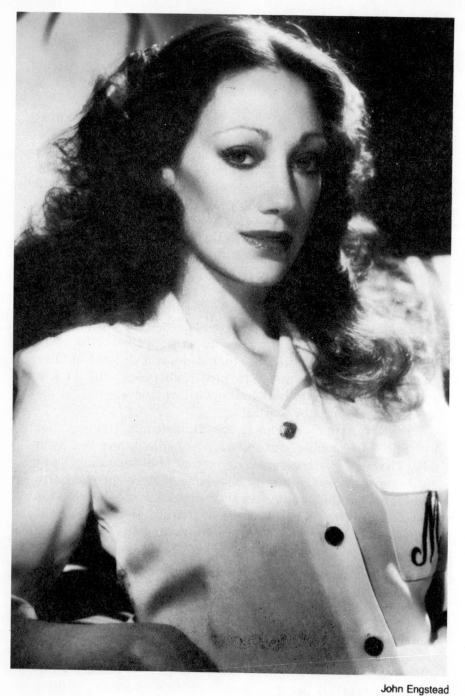

John Engstead

*"To me a spiritual connection with oneself . . . is much
more important than the physical or the pursuit of beauty."*

my being. I have never in my life been interested in planning more than one day to the next, but now there is a continuum to my life. This child. This extension of my self."

Always intensely spiritual, this new Marisa is nearly surreal in her detachment, her otherworldliness. As we talk, she is at times so vague as to be unreachable. There is no middle ground here. One finds her either completely entrancing, or completely unfathomable. We can manage only glimpses into her complex personality, as through a psychological swinging door. She is clearly a woman one beholds but cannot enter into. Marisa is still the girl who can perform for the camera while singing to herself.

We ask about her sense of self. She is certainly the most intensely spiritual woman we will interview. Does she believe that her physical beauty is influenced or determined by her soul?

"I have always had an intense belief in the spiritual . . . in God . . . in the basic goodness of life. I was raised in the Catholic Church but, as I grew older and more inquisitive, I began to search for answers in my own rather special concept of spirituality. I have faith in the intrinsic rightness and continuance of life. To me a spiritual connection with oneself, self-love, is much more important than the physical or the pursuit of beauty. Happiness comes through spiritual understanding. Beauty and peace of the being . . . of the inner self . . . of the soul . . . that is worth finding in life. That above all else."

Beauty of the soul. Perfection from the inside out. Marisa, the woman of thirty, is still the girl in front of the mirror, searching her reflection for spiritual understanding. Was it her soul she saw that day? We will never know. But it pleases us enormously to know that more than ten years later she still radiates the positive joy of living. The flower child is still blooming in Beverly Hills.

MAKEUP:
Marisa Berenson

MARISA HAS A perfect oval face with pale grey almond-shaped eyes, a distinctive nose, translucent ivory skin and a generous, sensual mouth. Although as she grows older it bothers her less and less, she feels that her nose is her least attractive feature and that her eyes are her best.

Marisa began using makeup in earnest when she became a professional model. By experimenting and watching other models she learned how to apply color and shadow and accentuate her remarkable eyes and classic bone structure. During her modeling years, her flair for dramatic makeup made her one of the most exciting women to photograph and caused her to develop a repertoire full of exotic techniques and styles. She was then, as she is now, truly a creature of fantasy.

Now, with incredible expertise at her command, Marisa has simplified her basic makeup to the barest essentials for day. She still, however, enjoys a reputation for looking outrageously beautiful with unusual makeup for evening, and her style remains uniquely her own.

Even for elaborate evening makeup Marisa spends no more than ten minutes on her face. She attributes this to years of practice and expertise. She makes up standing in front of a

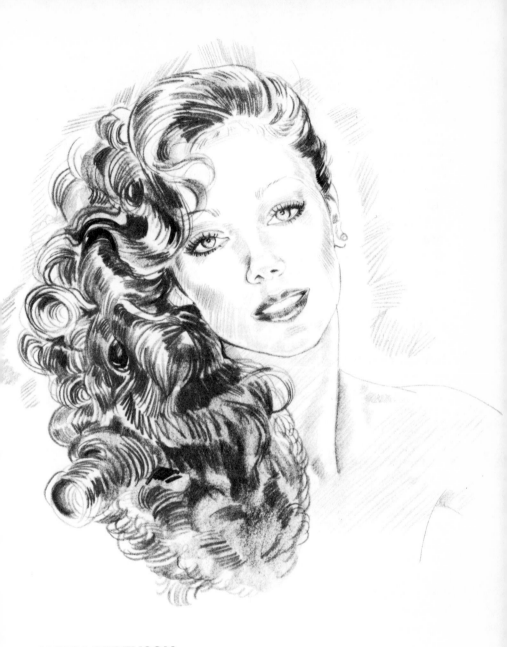

MARISA BERENSON

THE BASE: *Ivory foundation. Soft contouring with cream blush to accentuate bone structure.*

THE EYES: *Deep, mysterious shadowing; heavy mascara; high, arched brows.*

THE MOUTH: *Clear, soft color.*

THE FINISHED LOOK: *Cool, pale, expert and extremely elegant.*

special mirror and dressing table, rapidly and skillfully applying a light moisturizer, water-base foundation, cream blush and translucent powder. She admits to owning many lipsticks, but has recently switched from darker shades to softer, clearer tones. All of her basic makeup goes on with her finger and her lipstick comes right from the tube.

Marisa's eyes are, without a doubt, her most extraordinary beauty feature. They have an exotic, far-away dreaminess that she enhances with the careful application of deep, softly colored shadows and creamy highlights. Marisa loves heavy veils of mascara (not the most natural look, but certainly dramatic) and she insists that it be waterproof and not run down her cheeks when she laughs or cries. She prefers Dior, the blackest and thickest on the market, and manages to remove it easily each evening with eye makeup remover pads, saturated in oil. She uses cream or powder shadows in a broad range of colors, so long as they are quiet and flattering without being in direct competition with her eyes. For daytime, a simple swath of soft color does the trick, while for evening or work she will carefully highlight the lid and the bone beneath her perfectly shaped brows. Those thin, elegant little arches fastidiously repeat the shape of her eyes and finish off a face that is portrait-perfect.

The Bath (versus the Shower)

"THE BATH is a ceremony . . . a very spiritual activity. Potions and essences and perfumed oils are all part of the ritual. Bathing is the most luxurious, sensual way to cleanse the body."

When Diane Von Furstenberg describes her bath, her dark cat eyes flicker with pleasure. She conjures up visions of Ingrès' "The Turkish Bath": scented, slicked with fragrant oils, wildly exotic. We picture it all, standing in the middle of her exquisite suite of bathing and dressing rooms with their cabbage rose wallcoverings and elegant fittings. "Diane in the Bath" . . . an Ingrès update.

Bathing, they will all tell you, is a luxury few working women can afford. To be properly accomplished, it requires *the soak* and *the scent* and the whole shebang. All this takes time—of which most of us have precious little. Yet seven out of the eleven choose to bathe rather than shower (Marisa bathes in the evening, showers in the morning); if not every day, then as often as possible. And they all make a pageant of it.

They put everything but the rubber duckie into the tub. Flower essences and essential oils were favorites, the sort you can buy in good sachet and potpourri shops like Cherchez in

New York. The real nonchemical thing. Real rose oil. Real jasmine. Lemon verbena. Rondelitia. Myrrh. The sachets are put in little gloves and attached to the faucet where they release just enough scent and essence into the steam. Some of them have slimming power (we suspect that they draw the excess water out of the body through the skin in some manner). Most smell divine. The oils are highly concentrated, so potent in fact that a single drop can perfume both the bath and the woman (and the room!) for hours. Used directly in small quantities on lightbulbs, essences will release their fragrance with the heat of the lamp and scent the house.

It's a fact that water is very good for the body, taken both internally and externally through bathing or soaking. Add a dollop of moisturizer and you can turn an ordinary bath into a facial for your body. The moisturizer will penetrate deep into the inner cell layers while you relax. Lingering in this sort of bath has very real physical and emotional benefits. Cheryl Ladd takes a fifteen-minute soak every evening before bed and after her shower. The purpose is not to clean but to meditate. Ooommmmmm-ing in a scented, moisturized bath unwinds her completely and helps her to sleep. Liv Ullmann reads in the tub. A tub full of bubbles and *The New York Times.* And for Phyllis George, a bath full of Norell bubble bath is the treat of the week. She regrets having time only for a quick shower on a day-to-day basis, but when she bathes, she really bathes. "It's heaven!" says Phyl.

Mary Tyler Moore wishes she could be the kind of person who luxuriates in the bath. She just can't spare the time. She showers. As do Jackie and Olivia. And all of the above use soap (horrors!) on their bodies, although Olivia does use a body moisturizer after her shower since her skin is very dry. Ann-Margret has a great tip for shower-takers. She perfumes immediately after stepping out. Then the skin is warm, the pores are open and the fragrance seeps in and lingers a long while.

The best bathing tips come from Margaux and Diane. Margaux uses a French bath product called Aqua-Vat which, when put into hot water, causes the bather to sweat and forces impurities out of the skin. Margaux swears it helps rid you of the flu, too. Either with this type of bath product or alone, swigging a glass of cold mineral water while you steep also will help you to sweat it out. A cold splash after such a soak is really a necessity. It will close the pores again and leave you feeling squeaky clean.

Diane's pre-bathing routine is fascinating. She dry-brushes her skin. Using a natural vegetable bristle brush (a loofah would work nicely too), she brushes off the dead cells from her skin before stepping into her tub. If you've ever used a loofah to stimulate circulation you know that this sort of activity also helps fight cellulitis.

The sybaritic soak. Having seen some of these bathrooms firsthand, we can tell you that the atmosphere would be hard to match at home. Ann-Margret's tub comes to mind. For a girl who can't take the time to bathe, it's an inviting little washbasin. Gray marble. Gold fixtures. With a couple of whirlpool outlets on each side. And sunken about five feet into the carpeted floor so that you could submerge your pampered body and dogpaddle your way to dreamland. Oh, yes, and it's tucked into a corner framed by two floor-to-ceiling windows with shirred ninon Austrian shades which when opened (as they were the day we were there) allow the bather an undisturbed view of Benedict Canyon and Los Angeles beyond.

Excuse us, but would you please pass the soap.

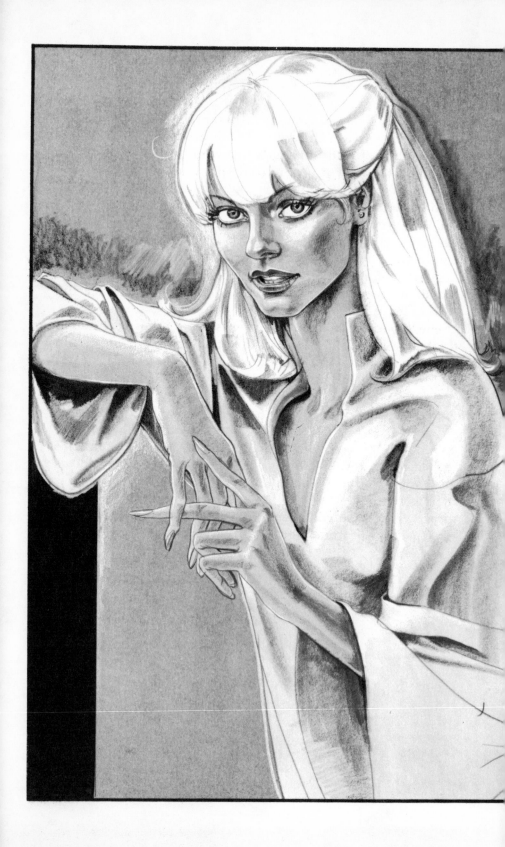

Olivia Newton-John

SHE SITS IN A fluff of sugar-water-stiffened crinolines and a dirndl skirt beside the freeway field of honor. Her tennies are white. Her socks are rolled. Her collar is the genuine Peter Pan article. She exudes girlish innocence.

She is, her expression confides to us, full of remorse. How can this modest vision of maidenhood *ever* hope to win the Black Knight away from ChaCha DeGregorio in her toreadors and tube top? ChaCha, who a minute ago bent herself neatly in half, her black ponytail to the ground as a signal to start the joust, while Sandy sat on the concrete abutment just looking on.

The movie, of course, is *Grease*, starring John Travolta as Danny Zuko and Olivia Newton-John as the ingenuous Sandy Dumbrowski. The virgin blonde. Sweetie in the white shoes. We surely aren't the first to wonder, but the question that comes to mind is . . . is Olivia Newton-John really "Sandra Dee"? Look at all those album covers, after all. All that sunlight streaming through corn-silk hair. Olivia in faded jeans. Semisubmerged in still waters (Do they run deep?) with flowers pinned over an ear. Scrubbed clean and shining bright. But just put that question to someone who's seen *Grease* (and who hasn't?) and he'll tell you that nothing that came before can prepare you for the Olivia who grinds John Travolta under the heel of her vixen red mules and romps through the funhouse in her black bustier and skin-tight capris in the final scene. Could this be the real Olivia? Is "Totally Hot" Liv, "You're the One That I Want," the very same girl who lulled away the pains of improper love in "I Honestly Love You"? She defies the tendency to pigeonhole.

Well, we wouldn't want to disappoint you. It really doesn't matter which Olivia you're rooting for. In the end, she is her own woman and, in all fairness, neither one of the above. There is about her, however, a very definite aura of sweetness, a delicacy and (if you'll pardon the use of a word out of style) a purity. She's very low-key. Very businesslike without ever being manipulative. Nice. She's very nice.

Let's begin at the beginning. It was one of those busy days when Olivia had such a short time slot for our interview that we were sandwiched between takes at the recording studio. She hustled over to the office of her recording manager, plopped behind a very uncomfortable executive-type desk, and apologized in advance for what would have to be a super-fast get-together.

She wore khaki green. Not your average militia-man ensemble from the local army-navy surplus store, mind you, but khaki nonetheless. Her trousers were rolled to just above her boots, her shirt was cream-colored silk, and the sweater was from Calvin Klein. She admits to having a preference for Calvin and Ralph Lauren, which is not surprising since their designs are tailored and low-key. Then she raises her eyebrows, smiles, and names Karl Lagerfield and the exotic Chloe, her real favorite. In any case, she looked perfect.

"Tell you about my makeup? Well . . . as you can see, I didn't have the time to put any on this morning. Awfully hectic today. (She turns to her friend and costume designer, a young Australian woman, and they both giggle a bit.) But if you'd like . . . if it would make it easier, I'll just put it on now so you can see for yourself. Let's see, now . . ."

She takes a small cosmetic case out of her handbag and un-

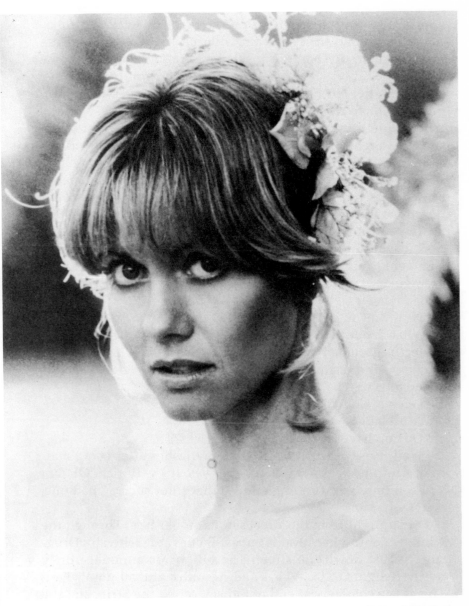

zips it, dumping the contents on the blotter. Not much, folks. A few tubes and little pots and a far cry from Ann-Margret's makeup table or Diane Von Furstenberg's veritable at-home cosmetic counter. She balances a little mirror from an eye shadow in her left hand and smudges, dabs, swipes—five minutes, complete with dialogue, and it's all over. Done. And the remarkable thing is that she doesn't look any different when she's through. You would swear she just stepped out of the shower.

Her makeup routine, like her surprising, spontaneous smile, suits her well. She is unstudied. She responds to our questions in the style of a woman who has been through this business hundreds of times. She's careful and measured and not, it would seem, given to rash judgments and ill-advised comments, but she never gives the impression that she's programmed. At times the honesty of her reactions surprise even Olivia herself.

"How do you get rid of unwanted hair?"

(What a question! Did we really ask this perfectly blond, perfectly groomed woman with the peach fuzz on her arms that *intimate* question?)

She blushes.

"I shave. God, did you ask everyone that?"

We all laugh.

"Do you have any special beauty tricks?"

"Well, I use a brush to separate my lashes after using mascara. And I use beeswax under my eyes. It's very rich. Oh, but you can only get it in England, so that's not such a good one, is it?"

The sunlight from the street settles on her face. Through the window behind her head is Sunset Boulevard. Schwab's Drugstore is just down the street. The billboards announce daily nonstop flights to Las Vegas and Acapulco and all points East. This is the commercial end of Sunset, called the Strip, and the traffic noises cause us to raise our voices slightly to be more easily heard. She is talking about Malibu and the horses she keeps there. How she exercises them in the Pacific surf. How she runs with her dogs. She appears to us to be intensely

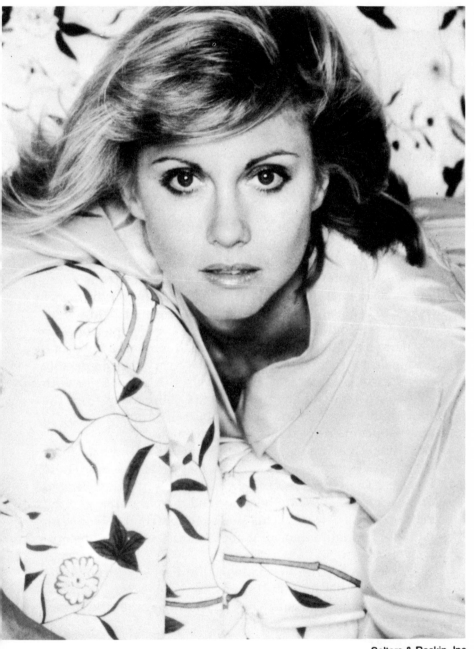

*"Having a life away from the public is all part of taking care
of yourself. And it's lovely to learn that people respect that
and understand!"*

private. She is talking with us but keeping a certain distance. It can surprise you, the moment when you first realize that she's left you behind. Olivia is sitting a few feet away from us, but she's only 45 maybe 50 percent here. The rest of her is in Malibu. That's better. None of the crassness of this neighborhood or the petty hustle of her busy day are getting to her. She's above all that.

"I used to be terribly afraid of the audience. You know, I'd walk out there scared to death. Shaking so I could hardly stand."

Her eyes get very wide and very blue. Her eyes are enormous. We hadn't noticed them before.

"But I'm over that now. I've learned to live with that fright and to really believe that people are there because they genuinely want to share with me. They're my friends and they're supportive. That's just one of the advantages of being well-known. I'm recognized now everywhere I go. People come up and talk to me. And everyone is so nice. It took me a long time to get over my stage fright. I am really a very private person. Lee and I would rather stay at home, just the two of us or with some close friends, than party. Having a life away from the public is all part of taking care of yourself. And it's lovely to learn that people respect that and understand."

Someone is pacing back and forth outside in the hall. Even with our backs to the door, we can feel them passing. There are voices. The vibes are very strong. Time's up, kids. Back to work. Back to biz. Back to the golds and the platinums and the American Music Awards. This sloe-eyed, peaceful person with the quiet of a Malibu morning about her is, after all, a recording star.

She is hastened into the hallway. On her way through the door she turns back and smiles at us.

"So sorry to have to run. They're waiting at the studio, you know. I hope I've been a help!"

Well, maybe not the red mules. And you can forget the sexy black top and the satin jeans. But, thank goodness, you can also cross off the white bucks and the circle pin. Olivia fits somewhere in between. A modest, hardworking, lovely girl whose life is just what she wants it to be.

MAKEUP:
Olivia Newton-John

OLIVIA NEWTON-JOHN'S finished makeup look could be an ad for Bonne Bell. It's what every young outdoorswoman should wear for a bareback gallop through the Malibu surf. She shines, she glows, she's so clean she squeaks. Olivia's makeup routine, like her life-style, is extremely low-key. And warmly attractive.

She smells like soap and water. She prefers to use cosmetics with no perfumes and, when she can, will choose the hypo-allergenic lines. Her skin is scrupulously cleaned, twice a day, with products from Aida Thibiant. She has facials at Aida's once every month or so and home facials in between. It shows. Her skin is healthy and beautifully clear. So clear, in fact, that Olivia never needs to use a foundation—just the lightest dusting of the sheerest powder she can find. Her favorite is from Alexandra de Markoff. When she needs a bit more color on her cheeks, she uses a gentle shade of cream blush from Clinique creams because her skin is dry and the Clinique creams hold longer. Olivia has a problem with fading colors. She says she can apply makeup and within half an hour it's gone. "The cheek stuff just sinks in somehow. And I don't know what happens to the lipstick. Could be I eat it off."

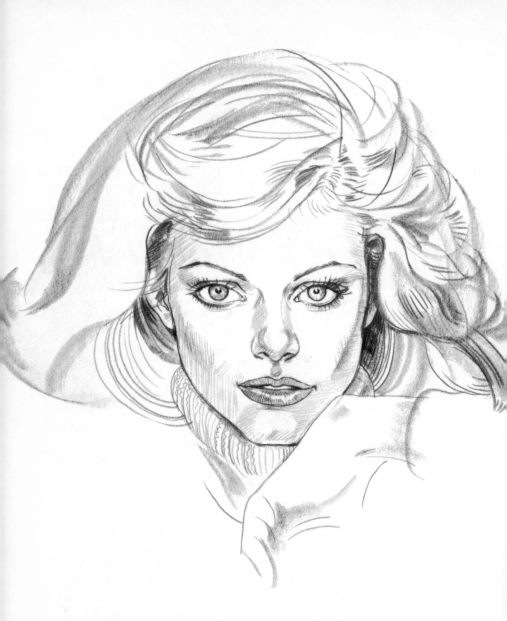

OLIVIA NEWTON-JOHN

THE BASE: *Clean, clear skin. No foundation. Cream blush in a soft shade on cheekbones. A sheer dusting of transparent powder.*
THE EYES: *Dark brown mascara, two applications, brushed in between. Neutral shadow for day. Mauve for evening.*
THE MOUTH: *Clear, natural gloss with a neutral-colored pencil outline.*
THE FINISHED LOOK: *Healthy, glowing, outdoorsy.*

Lipstick is not a hot item for Olivia. Forget the way she looked in *Grease*. Red never adorns her lips. And neither does much else in the way of colored lipstick. Her favorite look is a clear, natural gloss (again from Clinique, Meadowflower Honey; or a ginger shade from Dior) which she will occasionally outline with a natural-colored lip pencil.

Olivia's eyes are the bluest blue you can imagine. And they are huge! Bigger than they photograph and simply dreamy. She will take the time to mascara and often will use a trick taught to her by the makeup artist from the *Grease* crew. Mascara once, then separate the lashes by brushing through them with a clean, dry spiral brush, then mascara again. They get long and full without clumping together. Those spiral brushes are hard to find. Boyd's Pharmacy on Madison Avenue in New York imports them from France. Of course, in a pinch, any small brush will do.

For gala occasions, Olivia will use a little kohl on her lids or, more frequently, a touch of soft mauve shadow. On the day we talked with her, she had a Germaine Monteil Misty Violet eyecolor pencil in her bag, but her normal daytime shadow is brown, if any. No special contouring or clever application. She just dabs a bit on the lids and that's that.

She is as natural, as uncontrived, as sunshine.

Facials and Cleansing

JACKIE SAT WITH her face turned into the light. Her skin was free of makeup, nearly transparent, the color of fine English porcelain.

Suzanne's cheeks had the color and glow of New England apples. Not even blusher could mask that healthy shining skin.

Ann-Margret enthusiastically lined up her very large collection of bottles and tubes. There on the table was the basis of her beauty routine and her incredible skin.

Beautiful skin. All of them had it. All of them did a great deal to keep it that way. And it came as no surprise to learn that most of them paid a great deal of money to ensure that their famous faces would shine, no matter how much or how little makeup they wore.

The truth is, there are no shortcuts to beautiful skin. Memorable complexions cost time and money. You might have been born with great skin, but it's a brutal fact of life that you can't keep it that way for long without consistent, day-to-day care with top-quality products chosen to suit your skin type and your life-style. Heredity helps. Diligence helps more.

There *is* an occasional pimple among the Superbeauties. The difference is that they have infinitely more than Clearasil to make it go away.

The bottom line is cleanliness. And not a soap and water routine. Scientific "lotion/potion" cleanliness. Treatment. Facials. Deep cleansings. Professionally obtained. Personally supplemented on a day-to-day, hour-to-hour program. And the best of everything. The purest, freshest creams. The best care. The most exacting skin analysis. The most individualized products.

Now, all this might sound like so much hooey, or a flagrant waste of money, or both. But we want to tell you that we came away believers. That is to say, we were convinced that how you *care* for your skin, infinitely more than the makeup you may or may not then use, is worth every penny and every minute you can afford to spend. The lowest common denominator of beauty is the skin. Not the hairstyle. Not the eyeshadow. Not the dress. But *skin*. Truly beautiful skin can put everything else in the shadows. We've seen it for ourselves and we're here to tell you it makes all the difference.

Who's behind Suzanne Somers' sunny face? Annie Francine Steinbach, a French-born, Rumanian-trained registered nurse and skin specialist whose happy clients include Diana Ross, Diahann Carroll, Peggy Lipton, Debbie Boone, Suzanne and scores of others. Annie treats them all herself, working alone, personally administering facials and treatments, mixing her magic potions client by client, in Beverly Hills. She believes in deep cleansing, preferring emulsions, which seem to seep more deeply into the skin, to creams. Although she emphasized that she is not anti-cream, she does feel that many women use too many and apply them without a real knowledge of their particular skin types. Annie says that no one has one hundred percent dry or one hundred percent oily skin. Each of us is a patchwork of both. Yet we tend to treat our faces as a whole rather than dealing area by area and correcting accordingly. Annie treats by nose, chin, cheek, forehead, temple— one little dot at a time. Her products are her own concoctions and the ingredients are natural—so natural, in fact, that some of them need refrigeration to remain fresh. If you were to open Suzanne's fridge you'd find a small jar of fresh-fruit-scented, orange-colored mask made from raw eggs. The yolk gives the cream its golden color. Once opened, this delicious-smelling cream must be kept in a cool dark place to preserve its freshness and consistency. Suzanne uses it in combination with a cucumber/mint cleansing emulsion. Annie's products contain either water or fresh fruit juices and the only perfume is the natural scent of the fruits. What she does not mention is that the cost of this little jar, according to Suzanne, one of her most satisfied customers, is a steep $50. This could be due to the batch-by-batch method of production, but certainly not to lots of advertising dollars. Annie doesn't advertise. Her clients do that for her. She will, however, answer any questions and prescribe treatments by letter. If Suzanne is a product of Annie's skill, she's a woman all women can trust.

Phyllis George has her Mario. Mario Caruso has cared for her skin for years. He understands the special needs of skin subjected to heavy camera makeup and hot lights. Phyllis has a facial at least once every two weeks in which steam and a cleansing or peeling mask are used. Her astringent is a calamine lotion Mario makes for her. He even mixes up a little lotion that, when rubbed into the spot, clears up a pimple in a day or two.

All of the products contain only natural ingredients. Phyl uses chilled witch hazel, for example, around her eyes to reduce puffiness and firm up the skin. She also has a great little trick for travelers. Anyone who does a lot of flying knows how drying climate-controlled cabin air can be. So Phyl boards the plane wearing as little makeup as possible, finds her seat, opens her bag and pulls out her cleansing cream. Off come the last traces; on goes a generous helping of moisturizer. Off dozes Ms. George. A prearranged half-hour before touchdown, a stewardess wakes her and Phyl puts on her makeup—just in time to deplane looking rested, fresh and dewy. You might be suffering from jet lag on the inside but your face will be glowing!

Jackie Bisset wishes she had time for facials and massage.

She spends personal time on her face and body, but the only professional attention she can manage these busy days comes to her when she's filming, where lots of pros are hovering around the set. Her favorite cleansing and moisturizing products are just as no-nonsense as Jackie. Kyle Lotion, available at most drugstores, doubles as a makeup remover and an under-makeup moisturizer. She also uses it on her fingers or sponge when she applies Panstick or pancake. This trick really works. We've tried it with several different types of makeup and find that moisturizer worked into the makeup keeps the finished face fresh and natural-looking hours longer. When Jackie's sensitive skin turns dry, she uses Lubriderm. And the only eye cream on her dressing table is Vaseline, which is also the only lip gloss Bisset ever uses.

Jackie and Marisa, both inveterate mascara users, swear by Eye-Q's for cleaning mascara off at night. Marisa, incidentally, is a soap and water cleaner. The soap is, however, straight from a New York dermatologist, not Procter & Gamble. Marisa finishes her cleaning with a light scouring, using a Buff-Puff from 3-M. These cosmetic pads slough off the dead cells and leave the skin shining and soft. A sort of at-home dermabrasion. She finishes with moisturizer applied over her entire face and neck and worked gently into the skin.

Margaux Hemingway cleans with yogurt. No kidding! Straight from the grocery store. For a super natural facial, she mixes a raw egg, honey and yogurt, slathers it on her face and lets it be for ten minutes. Way Bandy taught her that one and she says it really works. She also will scrub from time to time with cleansing grains. Her skin can take it and, at times, needs a drastic cleaning to get the makeup she wears for film and photography out of her pores. Sometimes her skin goes "berserk" and she breaks out. Good cleansing and frequent facials keep it under control.

Suzanne has her acne troubles, too. It began when she was twenty-five. When it gets to be a real problem, she goes on antibiotics. Cheryl Ladd, who can also come up with a "button" or two, finds that soaping her face with Neutrogena after using her cleansing cream helps to keep the oil under control.

And Liv Ullmann says she wishes she could live on a mountain so that she could wash her face and body in mountain stream water. "You just feel cleaner when you use soap and water, I think." But knowing that tap water isn't that pure, Liv opts for Clinique cleansers and astringents. Her favorite method of deep cleaning has always been and always will be the sauna. She does the whole thing: the sauna and the ice water plunge.

Olivia Newton-John offered the most unusual tip. English beeswax. She puts it under her eyes as a supersaturated, super-rich moisturizer. Only a little is necessary, fortunately, because it's sure not available at your corner drugstore. Olivia's list also includes more readily available items. She'll use Oil of Olay and Noxzema from time to time, fitting them into her regular group of products just so her face doesn't get bored.

Ann-Margret believes that you don't have to be rich to be beautiful. She has a sixty-nine-year-old Swedish friend who has the skin of a fifteen-year-old; she cleanses regularly, eats good food, uses good sense and buys products from the five-and-dime. Ann-Margret's own product selections are less affordable. When her eye area is looking a little red at the rims, she goes on a ten-day Orlane B21 diet. She claims never to have found a better concentrated eye-treatment cream. She also uses a mineral water spray to set her makeup, a wonderful idea—especially in hot weather when loose powder can keep down the unwanted shine but tends to look pasty. Mineral water sprays give a healthy glow without disturbing the powder sealer. Ann-Margret's daily routine consisted of the products and the treatments she paraded out for us to see. Those little jars, bottles and tubes came from one of the best skin-care experts in the country, Aida Thibiant.

This wasn't the first time we heard the name Aida Thibiant (pronounced Ida Tibiant). Olivia also goes to Aida and uses all of her products; so do Ali McGraw, Marsha Mason and Marisa (from time to time). A freelance writer we know from New York flies out to see Aida on a regular basis and there's even talk of women who commute from Europe for a facial and cellulitis therapy. Our curiosity was aroused. We decided to pay her a visit and see for ourselves.

When we walked through the unpretentious doors of the Aida Thibiant Salon on North Canyon Drive we were buzzing with anticipation. Who could know what famous face would be in there, swathed with warm terry towels being sloughed and buffed to perfection. Whose voice would we hear coming from the next dressing booth? We waited awhile in the sunlit reception area, trying to look casual. The walls are the color of ripe apricots, very fresh and clean, and the general ambience is low-key and extremely quiet. There are no hair-dryers here. No rock-and-chatter. No Muzak. The silence was the first surprise. Aida herself was the second. Our own unfamiliarity with such gismos as hydrothermatique baths and the like had caused us to expect, perhaps, a blond Venus on wheels, laden with goop and gels and frantically enthusiastic. Aida is a petite, gentle, soft-spoken and extremely knowledgeable woman. She is not gorgeous. She is very likeable. And you trust her. Immediately. She and her trained personnel are warm and friendly, but there is a decided feeling of no-nonsense in the tiny treatment rooms. No sleight of hand. No razzle-dazzle. And when Aida herself gives you a facial, you understand what the excitement is about. The lady has magic hands. And magic creams. Everything smells of roses. Almonds. Rosemary, bay and lavender. Your skin is bathed, soothed, stimulated. It is *divine*. And her advice was so sensible, so reasonable and down-to-earth, we resolved to make it a daily credo.

"The whole purpose of my facials and the products is to clean. Cleanliness is primary. There are certain things you must always do, and others you must avoid. First of all, clean the face scrupulously two times a day. Never use soap. Soap is alkaline and it dries. Many people don't like heavy creams because they are difficult to completely remove. Our cleansers are water-based and very, very light. They emulsify the dirt without disturbing the natural oils of the skin. Then the Tonique, which is not an astringent and contains no alcohol, removes the last of the cleanser. Ann-Margret uses the Collendula cleanser and the Tonique Rafraîchissant Peaux Grasses."

The cool liquids are washed across the face as she talks. They smell of roses and mown hay. "If you need to clean with a scrub, never pull the skin. Always use a circular motion or, if your skin is not too sensitive, a little facial brush that rotates across the skin." Buzzzzzzzzz. The electric brush gently whirls across the bridge of the nose, under the chin. The air around our face fills with honey and almonds and a hint of licorice.

"Now for the steam." A little machine is turned on and within seconds a light, warm steam is directed toward the face. Having had our face steamed before, it is surprising how gentle and moderately hot her steam process is.

"The steaming is very carefully done here. Not too hot, not too close. Putting a towel over your head and standing over the teakettle is the worst thing you can do to your skin. If your skin is at all sensitive, you will break the little capillaries by doing this. Women who use the facial saunas or steamers at home must take care that the steam is not too strong or too hot, especially women with troubled skin. Too close and you can actually aggravate the condition. Now the pores are open. I will now sterilize the skin with a mild electric current called the High Frequency. You will feel nothing more than a slight tingle."

She moves a little wand with a dancing blue light back and forth across the face. The slight odor of lightning of ozone.

A silent assistant adjusts the soft terry towel around the hairline to protect the hair from the creams. Aida is talking and stirring, selecting the appropriate ingredients for the massage. "Your face is now perfectly clean. When the skin is cleaned in this manner, it breathes. The natural oils are stimulated to lubricate it naturally. And the skin is more receptive to the treatment creams. It glows. It is no longer sallow and colorless. No makeup can accomplish this."

Her gentle voice with its lilting French accent coos us into total relaxation. She begins the massage. Her fingers fly ever so lightly. But no matter how quickly they move, the skin remains still beneath them. "The skin is elastic. And like elastic it will stretch only so far and then it will go slack and limp. Even if the massage is *fort*—how do you say, strong—I never stretch the skin. I use circular movements only, working the treatment creams and the gels gently into the inner layers of the skin."

Bliss! May this never end. The advertising line from Orlane products flashes across the backs of our eyelids. "Why the rich look different from you and me." We would if we could buy this feeling every day of our lives!

"I will now apply the masque. Your skin is slightly dry so we have prepared a Masque Essentielle, made from *les herbes de Provence* . . . from bay leaf, rosemary and lavender. Ann-Margret uses this too, by the way. But since her skin is dry on the surface but quite oily beneath, she uses it in combination with Savon Dermatique, a special cleanser with camphor that relieves the oil congestion of the inner layer. Now you will rest for fifteen minutes while the masque does it work."

The silent assistant raises our feet and places another warm towel across our legs. Wrapped, warm, sweetly scented from the masque—in the darkness it's very womblike and primal. We drift off into a quiet mental corner. Fifteen minutes pass. Aida returns.

"Now the masque is rinsed away with the Tonique. A spray of mineral water to refresh . . . moisturizer . . ."—she gently massages the moisturizer into the face—"and, *voilà!* We are finished."

Undone. We are positively undone. There are no adequate words to describe this. A purely female experience. Well, that's not true anymore, is it? Now men have facials. But like this one? Being touched, manipulated with fingers, scents, lotions. It is all too sensual for words. And yet, terribly scientific at the same time.

"Did you know that we give body massage here now? The very same, but for the entire body. It is very relaxing and beneficial to the skin."

Sign us up! It's enough to make you delirious!

Several minutes later, we stand at the checkout counter, surrounded by our own little pink and green bottles and grey tubes. The bill is the equivalent of one's week's groceries for a family of four. We don't care. We'll live on Campbell's tomato soup and crackers for a month if necessary, but we will not leave without our bottles. They will fly in their own little Aida Thibiant shopping bag at our feet, not in baggage where they might be misplaced or broken. Total indulgence. We will not let the experience disappear. The scents from these bottles, these magic bottles, will bring it all back two delicious times a day.

There is a moral to this story. Months after our return to New York, friends are still asking what it is we've done to our skin. "You look so clean! Your skin is so clear!" No kidding! *It worked.* It still works. And, perhaps most important of all, good habits are being formed. The products, as effective as they are, are not as important as our new way of looking and dealing with ourselves.

Phyllis George said, "Until six years ago I just didn't think about my skin. Then one day I realized—hey, it's the only one I have. And I'm not getting any younger. The time is now."

Good advice, Phyllis. For all of us.

Phyllis George

"MY FIRST THOUGHT WAS, I can't believe it! It can't be happening! When you want something so badly, it's hard to believe it's real when it happens. The cameras zoomed in. I had to stand up, get out of that chair. One hundred million people were watching me on national television and I was paralyzed. Someone put the robe around my shoulders. Someone pinned the crown on my head and handed me the roses and the scepter. I heard Bert Parks say, 'Take your walk.' My legs wouldn't work. Then, somehow I managed to walk down that endless runway feeling like Cinderella at the ball. 'There she is!' Here I am! Little Phyllis George, the tomboy from Dane, Texas— Miss America!"

She still is. Phyllis George really *is* Miss America. She is wholesome and friendly and exactly the girl you'd want your brother to marry. She manages to stay down-home nice and dazzle you at the same time with a style and a smile that are genuine and heartwarming. She will, for instance, kiss you goodbye. And thank you for coming. If you like Phyllis on the tube, you would love her in person.

She's Texas, all right. One hundred percent. She'll tell you that the real natural beauties are the Texas girls and reel off a

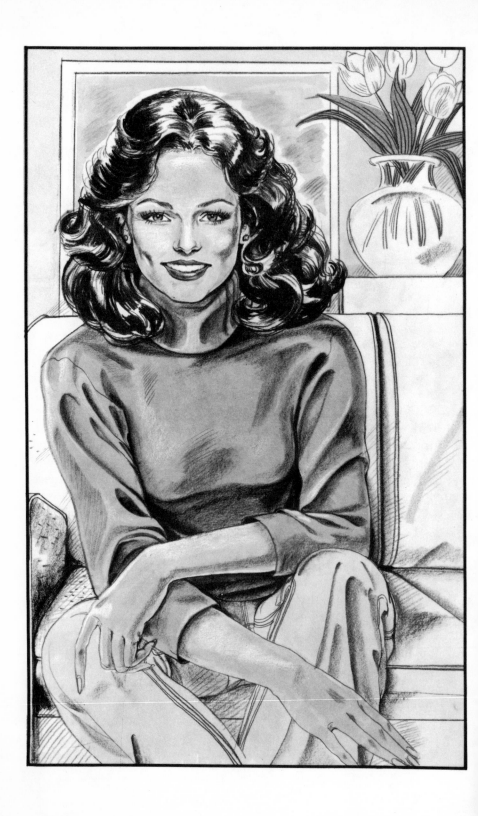

list of them including Susie Blakely, Farah Fawcett-Majors and Jaclyn Smith. Her own name is conspicuously absent. She's also modest about her beauty. Her good looks, like her personality, are straight from the shoulder, and when she flashes all those perfect teeth and that mile-wide smile, she's a wall-to-wall rainbow.

But what we like best about Phyllis is her sense of humor. She loves to laugh. Even at herself.

"As I walked down the runway, I nodded to the judges. And the *crown* fell off! It toppled right off my head and rolled down the runway. It was the first time in the history of the Pageant that had ever happened. Of all the luck! I guess I expected that somebody would pick it up, but when no one did, I just leaned over—on national TV—and grabbed it. Klutzy Phyllis! When I did that, of course, the robe slipped off my shoulders and I had to sort of tuck the roses and the scepter under my arm so I could carry the crown. My hair was sticking out from my head in two little horns where the crown had been pinned on.

"What a sight I was! A vision of American beauty and womanhood, and I dropped the crown! Everyone was choking with laughter. I didn't know whether to laugh or cry. But it did break the barrier between the image of Miss America and the person I really was. Everyone could relax and see that I was just Phyllis, after all. There was such sympathetic good humor coming up at me from the audience. You could almost hear them saying, 'Bless her heart. Miss America, a real girl after all!' "

Lights! Pathos! Cheering! Crying! She was born for it. Phyllis loves it. Every minute! There were a few mighty big drawbacks, though. When she talks about her life as a beauty queen, you can sense the discipline and determination that kept her going during the long year after that blockbuster evening in Atlantic City. The job of being America's sweetheart doesn't end on that runway.

There was endless travel. And the requirement that you look your best day after day, seven days a week, 365 days of the crown-toting year. Your makeup and your figure and the way you smile become your business venture. To this day, if you turn a camera on Phyl, the smile instantly appears. It's a habit she'll never break. She tended to herself like a prize filly, always grooming for the Derby. And she was tended *to*, surrounded by consultants. Consultants for her hair, her makeup, her diction, till she was "consulted to *death*." And she was photographed incessantly. Cutting ribbons, signing autographs, accepting keys to endless towns and cities. When this happens to you, of course, for the rest of your life you're followed by the popular notion that your every success, whether personal or professional, comes to you solely on the basis of your beauty. "I know people *look* at me. What I want is for them to *listen* to me!" It doesn't seem like a lot to ask that your mind be taken as seriously as your physique. Phyllis is, as are most Miss Americas, an intelligent girl with a college education and a good head on her shoulders. Being taken seriously is a problem she deals with even now.

"I remember so clearly that even when I was growing up, people would judge me on my looks and not on what was inside. There were always girls who were jealous of me and the attention I would draw. I was a cheerleader, the Homecoming Queen, fraternity sweetheart, sorority this or that. I loved it! It was exciting to be such a big part of the fun. But it caused a lot of envy and that bothered me. The nicest times were when I got a chance to talk with people I didn't know well so I could get to know them a little better. When it happened they'd say, 'Hey! You're just plain nice! You're really just a nice person!' That was the biggest compliment of all and the one I worked for the hardest.

"I learned an important lesson from those experiences. It may be your good looks that attract people to you initially, but the inner you has got to be beautiful to hold them and make them your friends. You have to get yourself and others *past* the outside. My mother has always said, 'Beauty is as beauty does.' That may sound corny but I've always believed it and tried to live my life by it. I never want to be known as just another pretty face."

She's not just another anything. She's one of a kind. Phyllis

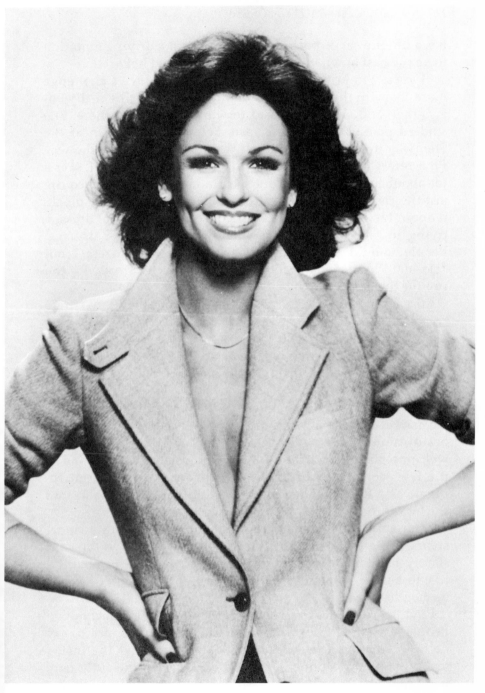

Harry Langdon

has a unique set of personal standards and a driving ambition to be the best at whatever she does. It's served her well.

"I guess I'm just a natural born achiever. I love a challenge more than anything!" Except winning, perhaps! She really enjoys that, and she's not afraid to work hard to get there. She studied piano for fourteen years before sitting down at the Steinway in The Competition. ("The Competition" is the way Phyl refers to the Miss America Pageant. That, in itself, says a lot about her.) She timed herself under sunlamps to acquire just the right amount of healthy, glowing tan—not too much, it doesn't televise well. She worried over her choice of dresses, trying to select clothes that would enhance, never upstage. People should never say, "What a gorgeous dress," but "Doesn't Phyllis look beautiful in that!" She was ready for the run for the title.

Miss Dallas, Miss Texas, Miss America! And then . . . there comes a time during that year of fame and travel when Miss America must ask herself, "What's next? Where do I go from here?" Not all of them have the desire. Few of them have had the right answer. Phyllis didn't hesitate. She knew what she wanted.

She chose one of the toughest, most competitive areas in the job market—professional sportscasting. It's a profession where beauty alone could never be enough. They don't toss out the welcome mat at the drop of a hankie. In fact, she was one of the few women who had the guts to try it, to use a microphone as a flying wedge to get her off that runway and into the locker room.

"The absolutely greatest thing about a job in professional sports is the thrill of knowing that, as a woman, you're constantly breaking new ground, you're completely unique. I'd like to be one-woman proof that commentators don't have to be men to be good!"

Phyllis just leaned over and grabbed the ball. Touchdown! People started singling her out at cocktail parties, not to say hello to America's favorite pretty face, but to get the inside scoop on Jimmy Connors, rub shoulders with the little lady who charmed the scowl off Muhammad Ali and lit up Joe

Namath like a night game at Shea. She quickly earned a reputation as a hard worker, a nuts-and-bolts performer and the respect of everyone who worked with her.

One of our sharpest impressions of her during her tenure on *NBC's Challenge of the Sexes* was a filming in Canada. She was up there to tape an ice-skating sequence. For reasons unknown, it was decided to continue even though it was snowing . . . and snowing . . . and snowing. Phyl stood there, looking positively Floridian, with her warm smile and twinkling eyes, all wrapped up in Russian lynx while everyone else shivered. She was pleasant, charming and unruffled as the snowflakes whipped around her head and Vince Scully turned blue. We asked her about that taping. Sure, she remembers. Who could forget? The windchill factor was below zero. She couldn't feel her feet. She nearly had to be carried away after the wrap-up. But, she hastens to add, it was much harder on the skaters.

Her concern for others is characteristic, as is her determination to succeed in spite of all the odds. What's a little snow to Phyllis? Or a personal setback or two? There were probably a few she didn't win on her way to the crown, too. She doesn't mention them. Setbacks are a nuisance, but—if you're real smart, and she is—you can learn from them. In any case, the eyes of Texas are upon you, so throw them a smile, pick up the pieces, tuck the roses under your arm, and keep going. She's come a long way from Atlantic City but, no matter where there's a competition, that's where you'll find Phyllis.

"Being Miss America was a wonderful experience for me. But I knew, even then, that I'd never let it end on that runway. I'm always looking for new things to do, new challenges, new people. You know, you should get a quotation from everyone's mother for the book, just to see if the person you're writing about has changed. My mother would tell you I'm just the same as when I was out to win that crown. Always working away, involved in twenty different things at once, never happy unless I'm busy heading *somewhere*. Somewhere I've never been before. That's the secret, that's what makes me happy, what makes me pretty. Can you understand that?"

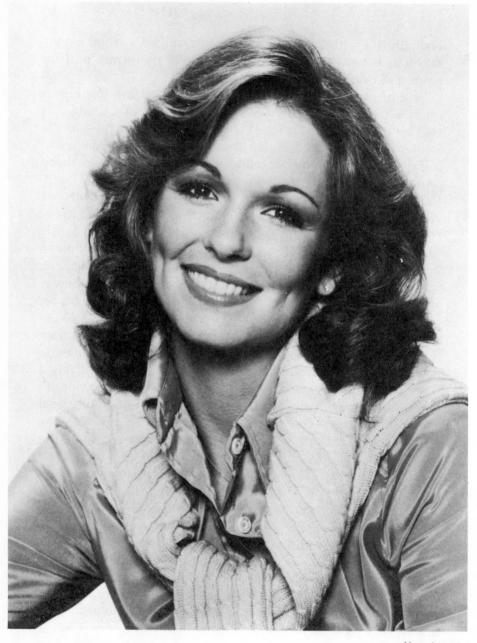

Harry Langdon

"Being Miss America was a wonderful experience for me. But I knew, even then, that I'd never let it end on that runway."

MAKEUP:
Phyllis George

WHEN PHYLLIS GEORGE first tried makeup, her idea of the absolute limit was an eyelash curler from Woolworth's. She still has it. Phyl is a collector, an experimenter, a creative whiz kid with the sponge, the brush, the tube and the jar. She's got one of everything on the market from each cosmetics company in existence. To Phyllis putting on makeup is just another way of having a good time.

Back in junior high, it was the curler. The finished lashes made her look like Betty Boop. She would finish it off with a giant glob of Vaseline on her lips. A little later on, she wowed the boys in Dane with her baby blue shadow and ruby red lips. By high school she was into foundation, eyeliner and a dozen different shades of lipstick. Her idea of Super Sunday was browsing through the latest issue of *Vogue* and *Harper's Bazaar* and checking out the photos of Suzy Parker. She took notes. She'd close herself up in the bathroom and try the look on for size, posing in front of the medicine cabinet mirror.

Then she went to college and graduated to false eyelashes. The bigger the better. You could never catch Phyl in Zoology II without her lashes.

When she became Miss America in 1971, she decided to cool

it. She put away all those bottles and lashes and glue and took a good, hard look at herself and her skin. With the help of Mario Caruso, a New York skin and hair specialist, Phyllis took stock and edited her routine. She also stopped copying the models in the magazines. She has discovered that Phyllis can look just like Phyllis and look swell.

These days her day-to-day makeup routine takes her fifteen minutes. No more. No less. For daytime she uses a lighter hand, for evening more intense color and more drama. What she's after in either case is a healthy, glowing look that is believable but not bare. To get it, she finds she requires a lot more color than most people. Her skin seems to drink up whatever is applied to it and within a few minutes after doing her makeup most of the color is gone. So she chooses good, strong shades and the result is bright and pretty.

Ask her to name some of her favorite products and the lists read like the contributing advertisers in *Vogue*. Revlon. Estée Lauder. Clinique. Elizabeth Arden. Maybelline. (If we've forgotten anyone, you can assume she hasn't.) For the girl who simplified her makeup style, she has a rather large permanent collection. She claims to own every shade of eyeshadow, even though her usual choice is in the brown tones. When she feels adventuresome, she'll try purple or pink with blue. And she owns every lipstick color made, cream and frosted, from pink to red to coral to peach to all the coordinate blushers. She loves to experiment with new colors, new combinations and new products. For Phyl, cost is not synonymous with quality. She'll pass the more expensive product and select the five-and-dime variety eye pencil if she thinks she can make it work for her and the color intrigues her. She's not predisposed to buy the expensive brands. In fact, in some cases she feels the only thing that changes between the two extremes are the boxes they're packed in.

Then there's the subject of application. Phyllis has more sponges on sticks, brushes and doodads than an illustrator. She prefers her own sponges, throwing the ones that come with the shadows and creams into the circular file immediate-

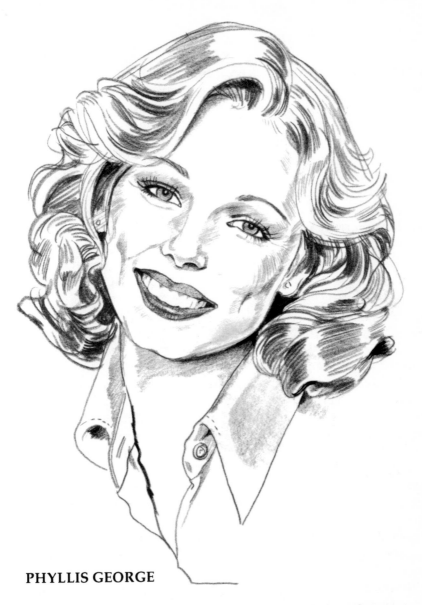

PHYLLIS GEORGE

THE BASE: *Light, sheer foundation. Contour creams in neutrals and colors to shape the cheekbones and diminish her dimples. Light powder to set.*

THE EYES: *Off-white powder shadow on the eyelid, contoured with a soft brown and blended. Dark soft pencil line above and below, near lashes, smudged. Black mascara.*

THE MOUTH: *Lip pencil to outline. Any one of dozens of colors of lipstick. Gloss.*

THE FINISHED LOOK: *Bright and healthy. Very careful and very pretty with emphasis on great color!*

ly upon opening the packages. She rarely uses her fingers because she believes that using fingers stretches the skin.

Does this give you the impression that she's having fun with makeup? It should.

Here are some Phyllis George tricks:

1. For eyes that look too small when you smile try using an off-white shadow on the upper lid and contouring with pale brown, just the way you'd do your cheekbones.

2. A dark brown or black line on both the upper and lower lids looks terrific when it's smudged into the lash line. Then mascara. It's a sexy, dark-eyed look.

3. Try a little brown or black eye pencil on the underside of the upper eyelid. It never looks like you drew it there and it fills in the spaces between your lashes. Then mascara.

4. Curl your lashes carefully. It takes forever to grow back a lash! If you have fragile lashes, try using cake mascara instead of roll-on. Roll-ons are faster but they have a tendency to dry out the lashes. Not so, the cake variety.

5. Lining your lips can make the difference between a smile and A SMILE. (Phyl has five different lip pencils to do the job, each a different shade. She then applies lipstick straight from the tube unless she's being photographed. Then she brushes.)

6. Dimples can be a liability if they're all you can see. Phyllis claims that hers make her look like a chipmunk unless she uses a contour cream. She contours with several shades, from her ears to the dimples, to brighten up her face and for balance. "Dimples are a deformity. It really blew my mind when I learned that. For years, kids at school used to say to me 'Here comes old dimple face!' They can take over your whole face if you don't watch out."

Phyllis also suggests that you use contour cream under your chin if you are an animated person and talk a lot. If you are, you might look a little double in the chin. (She found out about this little detail from watching herself on the tube!)

And, of course, contour if your face is too round. She does. "I had the cutest little puppy face you've ever seen back when I was Miss America. It's a bit better now. As you age, *everything* settles! Even those big cheeks!"

Phyllis really enjoys makeup. She has a great time playing around with colors and products. But she never looks overdone. That takes practice. We wonder if she still flips through magazines, looking for the latest beauty, and if she chuckles when she finds herself pictured there!

Manicures and Pedicures

PHYLLIS GEORGE NERVOUSLY checks her watch. She can't, she explains, be late for her manicure. Marisa Berenson moves her hands very slowly, effectively causing every eye in the room to focus on her inch-long, perfectly matched, deep red nails. Mary Tyler Moore mirrors her moods with color selected from the dazzling array of polish bottles on her manicurist's tray. And Suzanne Somers laughs aloud and admits that the secret to her long, tapered and totally natural fingernails is that she never, never does the dishes.

Anyone who doubts the reality of movie star hands has never been around these women. Sure Margaux Hemingway used to bite. Diane Von Furstenberg files hers down to nonsnagging squares, and Jackie Bisset will go to town on her garden and forget her gloves, but they all agree that unsightly hands are the kiss of death to a beautiful, pulled-together appearance. In their opinion, you can cut the dress, dear Scarlet, from the velvet drape, but your hands will tell on you.

In nail-conscious circles, the way to grow is with the wrapped, or Juliet, nail, a professional technique using tissue and glue. Once a week the manicurist cuts tissue paper in the shape of each individual nail and glues it in place, turning the edges under to give the entire nail surface an "outer skin" of thin but strong paper. This time-consuming procedure reinforces the natural nail, protecting it from splitting or chipping while allowing it to grow normally. The wrapped nails are then polished with two or three coats of color and sealed. If the polish is removed between wrappings, it is rubbed off from the quick up to the tips rather than the other way around in order to leave the wrap intact. When performed by a pro, this technique is both effective and invisible. When Phyllis George blows a kiss to the viewing audience, not a soul can see her wraps!

Phyllis, as a matter of fact, makes a "fetish" of her nails. Having lived with "the nubbies," as she calls them, for years (perhaps as a result of all those piano lessons), she admits to taking excruciating care with her hands. She, like most of the women interviewed, has regular manicures and pedicures; between appointments works on her nails herself, filing with a nonsnagging metal file rather than an emery board, cleaning up her cuticles with Revlon's Creamy White Cuticle Remover, and soaking her fingertips in olive oil to soften the cuticles and replace the moisture loss caused by polish removers.

Phyllis even admits to using human nail transplants! Unlike the plastic synthetics from the five-and-dime which have a nasty tendency to fall off into the soup, or the salon type which are thick and unsightly in profile, the human transplant looks one hundred percent natural when glued on to the real nail, allowing the nail to grow out underneath. The thought of sporting someone else's fingernails may seem a bit unhygienic, and Phyllis didn't fill us in on the methods for *harvesting* donor nails, but the effect is intriguing.

Marisa Berenson, whose nails are downright unbelievable, has a favorite manicurist. The fact that she works at Carita in Paris doesn't seem to cause Marisa a problem, even though she sighs and regrets that she doesn't get to her too often these days. She goes to a more convenient salon once or twice a month for the works, agreeing with Phyllis that even in winter, a good pedicure, although invisible to the outside world, makes all the difference. Marisa's nails are so long that the color of her polish has a very definite effect on her outfit. The day we visited her, her nails perfectly matched her bright red oxfords and precisely repeated their patent leather shine.

Mary Tyler Moore's husband, Grant, whose opinion Mary welcomes in most matters, disagrees with her on the subject of nail length and color. "Grant hates long nails painted in bright colors," she says, "but I feel that they lengthen my hands and add to my femininity." Even in her most frivolous moments, however, Mary will not reach for the blood reds and purply shades at her manicurist's table. She prefers the clean, clear reds and cheerful russets. To brighten up the shine between manicures, she adds another layer of top coat. And she makes sure that, although beautifully shaped, her nails are kept at a manageable length. Her straightforward approach to length and color suits her no-nonsense style. Mary's nails would never interfere with her firm, warm handshake.

On the other hand, we have Margaux Hemingway. Nails just aren't Margaux's strong suit. She keeps them short and simple and unpolished. She will even take a bite or two under pressure. Though "The Babe" speaks for a nail polish company through its perfume line, she's too outdoorsy to cultivate glamorpuss nails.

Nor will you see polish on the delicate hands of Olivia Newton-John. That's just not the nature of the girl who rides her own horses through the Malibu surf. Natural is. Healthy and buffed with no artificial additives.

Olivia and Margaux are two of the naturalists. Cheryl Ladd also has healthy nails with pink pinks and white whites and a no-fuss look so few of us can ever achieve without splitting and tearing. And for Diane Von Furstenberg, with a business career in the garment center where she handles fiber, particu-. larly synthetic fiber, all day, short square nails are the only answer. Liv Ullmann's hands are so expressive that color on her nails would only detract from their beauty. So she doesn't bother. But please don't be misled by this seeming casualness. Even though all of the above prefer unpainted nails, and some prefer short to long, none of them have ragged cuticles or nails torn to the quick. Nearly every one uses a professional manicurist. Hands count among the beautiful, no matter how offhanded they may sound!

Our favorite hand story, however, comes from the honest and witty Jacqueline Bisset. Forever British, Jackie *loves* her garden. It has remarkable curative powers when she is between films, exhausted and in need of a physical release. Out she goes into the brutal Los Angeles sun to weed or dig. Suddenly, in the midst of cathartic rooting and tearing, she looks down at her hands and discovers she has forgotten to wear her gloves. Again. "My God! Are these the hands of a movie star?" She stands there puzzling over the best course to take. Go in and get the gloves and spoil the delicious feeling of the earth on her naked hands? Or wait until she begins to work and worry about getting her nails in shape for the camera. "What the hell," she sighs. "I'm too busy living to be beautiful now!" If Bisset's beauty has been seriously affected by her green thumb, so far nobody's noticed.

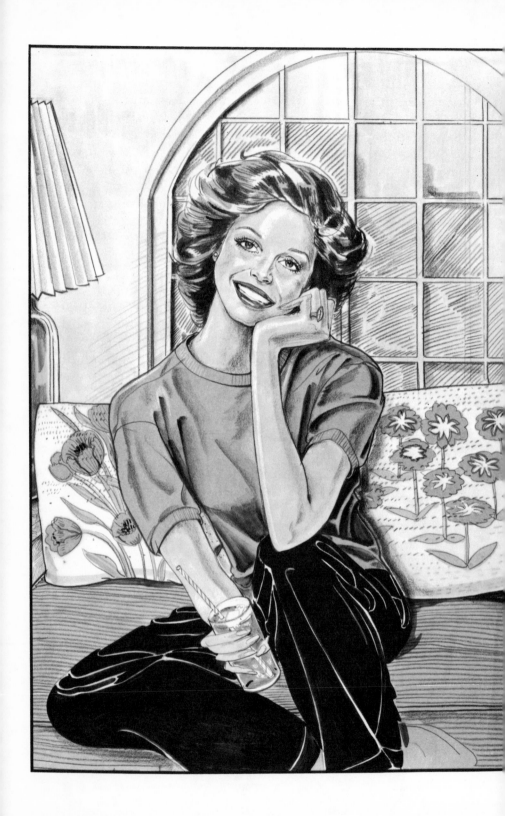

Mary Tyler Moore

WHEN MARY TYLER MOORE listens, she really listens. She looks you straight in the eye and gives you her complete attention. She makes you feel brilliant and witty—as if you were one of the most interesting people she's met in ages. And should you compliment her on something, she says thank you with such spontaneity you know she means it. She's genuine and responsive. That ability to listen and respond are qualities that pervade her personality and her acting, and have turned millions of strangers into ex-officio members of the MTM Fan Club. People like Mary because Mary likes people and it shows.

We spent nearly two hours with her, and one of our most lasting impressions was that everything Mary does or says is appropriate. Never formal or simply polite, but perfectly in keeping with the situation. And in someone as busy and successful as she, that is quite an accomplishment. You feel as if you could enjoy her for years without any discomfort. Her six-year run as Mary Richards is proof of this. And Mary Richards, she says, was a character she played close to her real self, letting her natural responses come through the role. Like that character, the real Mary takes that little bit of extra time to really relate to people, rather than simply passing time with them. She has a niceness about her, a warmth. You are comfortable right away. She extends her hands, shakes warmly, offers you lunch, something to drink. She smiles. She laughs at your jokes. *She* compliments *you*, encourages you and helps you to do your job better.

Another thing you notice right away is that Mary is a very private person. She talks about her professional life with professionalism and about her personal life with great care. There are things she won't discuss. She won't, for example, name any specific products because she feels doing so would mean making endorsements as far as the general public is concerned and she is "not in the business of making endorsements." Immediately you understand that this has nothing to do with being paid for endorsing a product. She simply doesn't do them and that's that. She really understands her media clout and how to use it effectively. When Mary Tyler Moore speaks out for or against something, millions of people listen. So she saves it up carefully for the things she feels strongly about—like Planned Parenthood and Save The Animals and diabetes. This tells a great deal about the level of her concern. It is centered on others, not on Mary.

About twelve years ago Mary learned that she had diabetes. She has, in typical fashion, completely adjusted her life to accommodate her condition. She takes insulin every day of her life. She watches her diet carefully. But she hasn't allowed diabetes to slow her down. In fact, she feels she has become a healthier person.

Now she exercises for more than her figure (exercise is a vital part of diabetes treatment) and is more aware of her general well-being. "I see to myself," she says. Her diabetes, like everything in her life, is under control.

She's a notoriously hard worker. There's nothing accidental about her success or her acting skill. She's been a worker all her professional life—doing it once, doing it twice and, ultimately, doing it superbly well. She's been at it for a long time. Mary started dancing at nine. She danced her way through a Catholic girls' school and then, two days after her high school

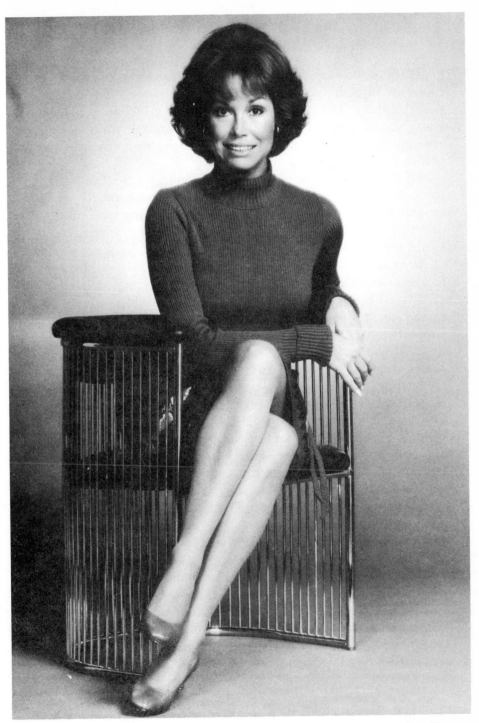

Tony Espanza

graduation, took her first professional job, a series of commercials. She says she knew, all through high school, that college wasn't for her. She had other things in mind and, like so many young people with a lot of ambition, felt there wasn't enough time to get a degree. This is something she now regrets.

"I had a lot of ambition and a lot of energy from the beginning. I decided very early that there wasn't much work around for chorus dancers. They weren't making many musicals. So I signed up with an agent who was just as ambitious as I, and we started making the rounds. I was lucky. I have one of those faces everyone feels comfortable with. I was the perfect girl next door.

"The enthusiasm was there from the beginning. The talent came later, much later, after a lot of hard work and experience. It's all a question of attitude. Set your sights high, believe in yourself and just get going. The talent, the skill, comes with the doing. Of course, there are some people who are born with it. Like Dick Van Dyke. He's a born genius. But most of us develop our skills as we go along. My biggest regret is that I didn't slow down enough back then to go to college. I really am convinced that a good education makes a big difference, no matter what you ultimately decide to do with your life. A fine education shows up in everything—the way you talk, the way you listen to people and respond to them, the way you do your job. The more you know, the better off you are."

Mary is a very self-aware person. Her familiarity with her public face comes, she says, from being able to watch herself, week after week, on film. It teaches her about herself. She has what she describes as a "friendly" face. "I am not a beautiful woman. I have a likable face, a face that's easy to live with. When I was younger, I hated my mouth. It seemed to me then that it took up my whole face. I was all mouth and teeth! Now, when the subject comes up, people tell me it's my best feature. I decided a long time ago that the best thing to do about something you don't like and can't change is to forget it. Get on with the more important things, like how beautiful you are on the inside!"

Mary lives in secluded Bel Air in a rambling, spacious, but by no means pretentious house with her husband of sixteen years, Grant Tinker. He is not there with her on the day we visit, but he is very much a part of her conversation. Pivotal, in fact. Mary is wildly in love with her husband. It shows in everything she says about him. He is the center of her life, both personally and professionally. What makes their long marriage even more remarkable in that split-up society is that they not only live together, they often work together. They are the principals of MTM Productions, which has turned out *The Mary Tyler Moore Show, Rhoda, The Bob Newhart Show* and many others. Grant, says Mary, is her best friend. He advises her, counsels her, gives her emotional and moral support, and is always there when she needs him. When something is on her mind, a personal or professional problem to solve, she consults Grant. Her face glows and her eyes light up when she talks about him. "The only way to describe my feelings about Grant is to say I'm madly in love with my husband!"

Listening to her talk about their communicating, supportive and loving relationship, we can almost visualize them here, sitting in front of the fire enjoying a drink before dinner and chatting about the events of their individual working days. It's a very pretty picture.

When the problems get bigger than the two of them can manage, however, Mary will seek out professional advice without hesitation. She feels that a good long talk with a psychiatrist, a sort of third opinion, can make all the difference when things get too tough. Anything that contributes to getting to know yourself fits her personal style. Analysis is a positive direction for anyone, she thinks. "Not," she hastens to add, "a major commitment to five years on the couch. Three or four visits may be enough to turn you around or help you decide." It's a healthy attitude and it works for her.

One surprising note: Mary hasn't got many girlfriends. She doesn't need them. Grant is quite enough for Mary. She feels that spending a day shopping with the girls, chatting over lunch at some fancy restaurant, gossiping or sharing confidences that exclude "the boys" are a waste of time. This is remarkable for several reasons, especially as Mary seems the kind of person who would relate beautifully to other women. She does, in fact. But she chooses to keep those friendships at a good distance from her day-to-day life and her marriage. She and Grant are a closed circle of two. Not even the children can penetrate their intimate rapport. Grant has four by a previous marriage. Mary has one, now a young man, a photography student long since on his own. She doesn't say much about the children except that she is a better career person than she was diaper-changer. The subject closes and we move on.

On to the subject of women and liberation. Mary is a strong supporter of the ERA and feels sympathy for the Women's Movement, except when it "hurts itself" by exaggerated actions or beliefs. "I'm for equality. I'm bothered by injustice to anyone and, as a woman in business, I'm all for being treated fairly. Equal respect, equal pay for equal work. It appalls me to read that there are only fifteen women in this country who earn $100,000 or more a year in business. That excludes the creative fields, of course. But it's grossly unfair! How many men do you think there are in the country who earn $100,000? It's time for those figures to even out. It's time for us. I'm one hundred percent for women."

Another injustice is the emphasis on youth, particularly in the case of women. "I see it all around. In the ads, on the fashion pages, on the screen. It's a big message in our society. Youth and beauty. It's very destructive. Beauty may change its form, but it's still there as you age. Oh, I believe in helping yourself stay attractive—coloring your hair if being grey upsets you. I've been coloring my hair for years now and I'm not ashamed to admit it. And I would have plastic surgery if it were important to me and I could afford it. That's just an extension of putting on your mascara, after all. But I hate to see women do these things out of a desire to remain young. Be the best you can be, at each stage of your life."

At the time of our visit, Mary was filming the Betty Rollins book, *First You Cry*. The portrayal of a woman who has had a mastectomy was both a gratifying and an unsettling experience.

"All of us, consciously or unconsciously, fear the possibility

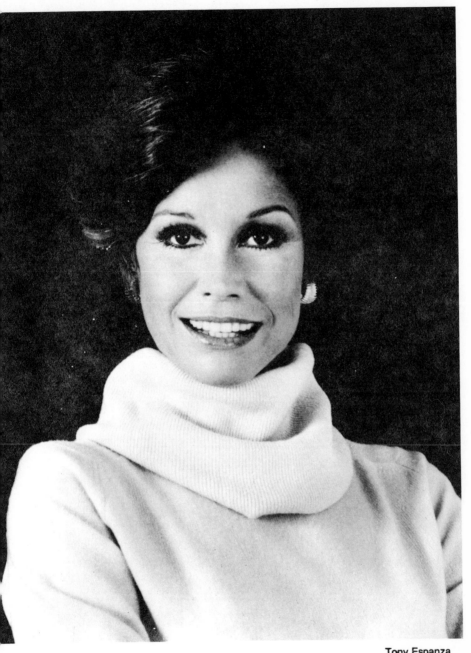

Tony Espanza

*"I have one of those faces everyone feels comfortable with. I
was the perfect girl next door."*

of breast cancer. Most of us are ill-equipped emotionally to handle the reality, should it be necessary. This illness strikes at our most vulnerable level of self-esteem, the loss of a part of our womanliness. It's interesting to know that researchers have discovered that it's the woman who has a difficult time resuming her sexual activity after the operation—not her husband or her lover. I sincerely hope that by doing Betty's story I am able to get her message across—to help women to understand the emotional side of the illness and be better able to deal with it if necessary. I know that the experience has been invaluable to me."

Self-esteem. Equality. The rights and the needs of others and the beauty of the individual. These are the real concerns of her life. Clearly, Mary Tyler Moore is much, much more than just another pretty face.

MAKEUP:
Mary Tyler Moore

MARY TYLER MOORE is all smile. On some, a grin that big would be a liability. On Mary, it's her biggest beauty asset. Why? Because she decided to make it just that. As a kid Mary hated her mouth. When she was fifteen and allowed her first touch of lipstick (but no eye makeup) she hated it even more. Her mouth was the first thing everyone noticed. It still is. But a long time ago Mary decided that it's better to smile your own smile than to spend your life trying to make your mouth look smaller. So she smiled. And the world smiled with her.

She does have a few don'ts about that mouth. She doesn't color it much. No matter what the current rage, Mary never uses deep reds or dark shades; only light, clear colors and only for special occasions. For day, she glosses or goes without. For sun protection, she'll use a sun screen or anti-chapping stick.

Another trick is the balancing act she plays with her eyes. Remember how enormous the eyes looked back in the late Sixties when lipsticks were very pale? And if the eyes are emphasized and the mouth played down, the mouth looks much *smaller*. So Mary does a real job on her eyes. For a reason she can't explain, her eyes will tolerate a lot of color without looking overdone. It has something to do with her bone struc-

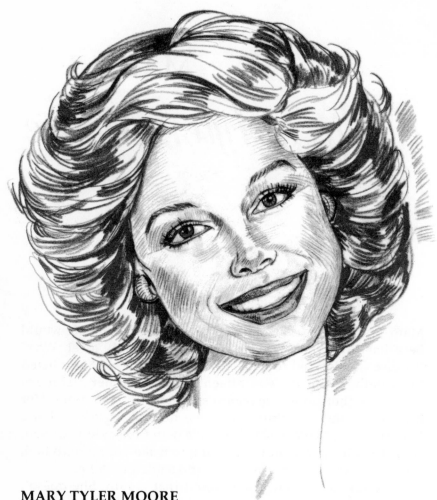

MARY TYLER MOORE

THE BASE: *No foundation for day. Contour cream in brown under cheekbone to give her round face some planes. Colored blush on cheekbones. Very little powder, if any, and only on trouble spots.*

THE EYES: *Taupe and grey shadows, used together and heavily, for emphasis. Penciled brows, brown mascara.*

THE MOUTH: *Nothing or next to nothing except on special occasions. Gloss or sunscreen.*

THE FINISHED LOOK: *Morning fresh and natural. No real effort to alter any feature through makeup, only through the lack of makeup. Healthy-looking.*

ture. Now, when we say color we mean neutral color, specifically taupes and greys in combination. Mary never uses blues or greens but she's heavy-handed with the neutrals. She clarifies her brows with an eyebrow pencil and mascaras with a roll-on. As a result, her eyes stand up to the prominence of her mouth—and her face balances.

As for foundation, Mary doesn't use it. She has a tan most of the time so, unless it's a very special occasion, she skips the base and moves straight to the shading. She adds planes to her round face with brown contour cream, applied directly under her cheekbones. Then she dusts on a little color blusher. She powders only the problem areas, like around her nose, and since her skin is basically dry she gets by without looking shiny.

If you were asked how many lipsticks she owns, you'd be right if you guessed a pair. Two. That's it. Once in a while she'll experiment with something new (like using lip pencil and no color, just gloss) but her biggest beauty hassles involve having a favorite color discontinued. She's loyal. Even though Mary wouldn't name names, everything she uses comes from an ordinary cosmetics counter.

She looks terrific. That little bit applied with skill goes a long, long way. She sums up her approach to making-up: "I want to spend no more than ten minutes a day and put on as little as possible and end up looking as if this is how I look when I get up in the morning. Real. Fresh-faced. And smiling." She does.

Health, Fatigue and Relaxation

"AND WHEN ALL ELSE FAILS, I . . ."
Make breakfast.
Go to Disneyland!
Play the piano.
Get up off it and exercise!
Take a bath.
Take a nap.
Meditate.
Read *Newsweek*.
Ride a horse.
Go to bed.
Vacuum.

What do you do when the camera crew arrives at seven A.M., the press conference is at nine, you leave for the studio at ten and shoot till noon, at noon there's an interview, another at one, a fitting at two, then a manicure and a pedicure, and you roll home at nine to a brand-new husband and a teenage child? What do you *do*, Suzanne Somers?

"I crash. I sleep. When all else fails and I'm strung out and cranky and insane from my schedule and the pressure, I just go to sleep. I'd suck my thumb if I could!"

We've got to admit, in a one-to-ten tension test, ulcer for ulcer, these gals have us beaten by a mile. The glamour girl with her hair in curls propped against pillows in a silken bed with a nail buffer and twenty pounds of raspberry cream is just not the scene anymore. They don't make 'em like they used to. They make them busier. They make them better. Not only are these women beautiful, they are beautiful under severe stress and with killer schedules. That in itself is an inspiration. They find time to fix a nail, find a dress, tint their hair and deal with their personal and professional problems in the midst of chaos. (And we have trouble coping with the week's shopping and labeling raincoats for the kids!) How do they do it? In a lot of ways, both funny and wise.

Suzanne not only sleeps a lot, she takes a lot of vitamins. The magic combination of in-bed-by-ten-out-by-seven and a multiple or two keeps her on her feet. When she's in extremis, really zonked, she'll nap in the afternoon. She figures she's alive today because she's basically a healthy person. Let's hope so. Because from time to time, Suzanne gets so busy with the filming and the this and the that, she forgets a few things. Like eating. She *forgets* to eat. That could singlehandedly destroy a person's stamina! Not Suzanne's, apparently.

Mary Tyler Moore guesses that she makes it through days like that because she 1) loves what she's doing and 2) enjoys physical well-being and 3) exercises (which helps in the well-being department!). She and hubby Grant tried meditating together a couple of years ago but they couldn't find the necessary forty minutes a day. As Mary put it, "We were getting more headaches trying to find time to meditate than we had before we meditated. In other words, we figure we weren't anxious enough." When Mary gives up in total frustration, she reads *Time* or *Newsweek* and tunes out.

Ann-Margret certainly has had personal and career problems to deal with in her time. But years and years ago her mother and father taught her when you have a fall, just get up again. And that's what she keeps doing. Over and over again. When she can't cope, she doesn't. She runs on the beach. She exercises. She gets up, gets out and spends time with others.

Anyone who could fall twenty-five feet from a scaffolding, then get back up there a few weeks later to sing and dance isn't going to be stopped by a run in her stocking.

Phyllis George has studied the piano for fourteen years. Now comes the reward. When Phyllis is bewitched, bothered or bewildered, she tinkles those ivories. Works wonders! She also reads. Everything she can get her hands on, she says, from *Time* to train schedules. She also takes vitamins and has regular checkups. But her ultimate weapon against stress and fatigue is her own brand of meditation. Round about five-thirty on long, hard days Phyllis sits down by herself and sorts it all out. She is a very organized person and tidying up her mind in this way gives her the confidence and peace of mind to jump back into the fray.

It takes a lot of nerve to ask Diane Von Furstenberg what she does to relax. You've got to be unrealistic to think that a woman who has built an empire out of a sample dress in a mere nine years has time to do anything at all. But we asked anyway. You never can tell. She bathes. Now that's creative relaxation. Combining the bare basics with the frills. Since she has to bathe anyway, Diane turns her tub into her hobby. She also runs away to the country over the weekend and walks, cooks, shows movies and, in general, goofs off. We wonder how many uninterrupted bucolic weekends she's actually enjoyed over the past few years. But then Diane is the sort who thrives on stress; you can see it in her eyes. "Pressure makes you strong," she exclaims in that sultry voice of hers. And when you've been watching the store for nine years straight without a single long vacation, you could turn into the "Man of Steel, Able to Leap Tall Buildings in a Single Bound . . ."

There are less demanding ways to weather the storm. Olivia rides bareback through the Malibu surf on one of her many horses. Liv Ullmann whips up a special Swedish breakfast or reads whatever magazines come to hand till she's back in control. Margaux Hemingway, who is one of the healthiest young women we've ever met, takes naps. She also likes to get a good night's sleep. All of the above in combination with whopping doses of vitamins and that unbelievable exercise program of hers keep her energy level in the top drawer. But Margaux's special weapon against the blahs is meditation. It pulls her back together when she's all bits and pieces. Meditation works for Marisa, too. That and her unshakable belief in God. That's got to be the most timeless solution and it's sure nice to hear about it. Cheryl Ladd simply closes the door on Cheryl, Career Girl, and throws open the one to Cheryl, Wife and Mother. She and David play touch football in the park with Jordan. Or ride the swings with Jordan. And sometimes Cheryl just pulls her hair back into pigtails, puts on a dumpy old dress and a pair of dark glasses, and the family runs away to Disneyland!

You are left with the tantalizing question, *Who vacuums?* We'll tell you this much. Her nickname is "Miss Hoover" because that's the first thing she grabs when the going gets rough, the schedule is killing, the phones are all ringing, her hair is unruly and she could just *scream.* She who vacuums the whole house, even under the rugs, doesn't look too domestic in a bikini—or in a Toque Blanche, for that matter. We're willing to bet that Jackie Bisset is the best-looking vacuumer on the face of this whole frantic earth!

"And when all else fails, I . . ."
Make breakfast—LIV ULLMANN
Go to Disneyland!—CHERYL LADD
Play the piano—PHYLLIS GEORGE
Get up off it and exercise!—ANN-MARGRET and MARGAUX
  HEMINGWAY
Take a bath—DIANE VON FURSTENBERG
Take a nap—MARGAUX HEMINGWAY
Meditate—PHYLLIS GEORGE, MARGAUX HEMINGWAY, MARISA
  BERENSON
Read *Newsweek*—MARY TYLER MOORE, PHYLLIS GEORGE,
  LIV ULLMANN
Ride a horse—OLIVIA NEWTON-JOHN
Go to bed—SUZANNE SOMERS
Vacuum—JACKIE BISSET (*who also weeds, but vacuuming was funnier!*)

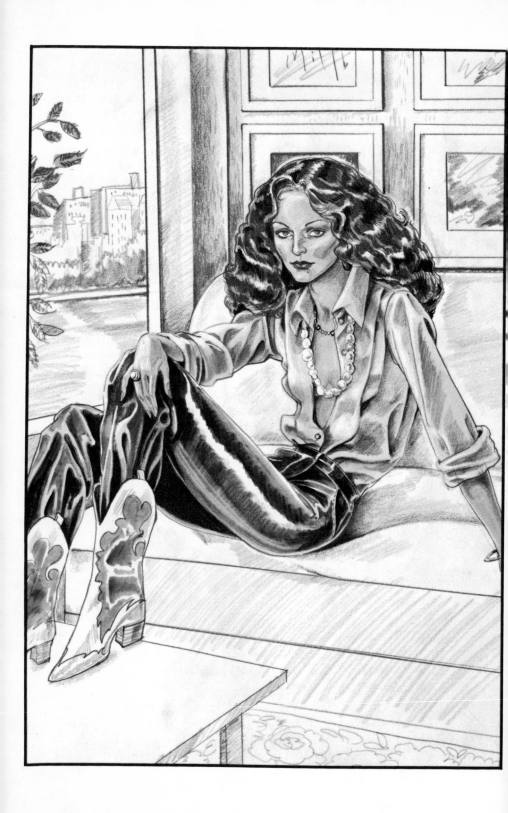

Diane Von Furstenberg

SOME SAY IT ALL BEGAN in a flash of brilliant merchandising. She singlehandedly brought back the dress in a market full of separates and blew the lid off the pantsuit monopoly. Others credit her prestigious name and a lot of string-pulling. Or her husband's endless money. In some versions the magazines spawned her, and the powerful and influential Editor-in-Chief of *Vogue* magazine, Diana Vreeland, was the deus ex machina. But to hear it told at *Vogue*, the girl with the highborn name and some samples in a suitcase was ushered in and out of that famous red office as through a revolving door. On Seventh Avenue scuttlebutt has it that it was her name alone that wrote the first orders. The question is, whom do you believe? How did Diane Von Furstenberg, ex-princess, become Diane Von Furstenberg, entrepreneur, in nine short years? Whichever version you choose, it's a great story.

Everyone in this highly competitive industry, fan or foe, admits that her timing was excellent. They'll also tell you it was intuitive. She certainly didn't have a retailing degree from the Fashion Institute of Technology. But then, anyone who was buying as much as she was had to have a good idea of what was missing. And what was missing was the little dress. Cut in simple, soft cotton jersey in nothing prints, and wrapped around the body in a way that flatters almost any figure from size four to size sixteen. That in itself was a stroke of genius. And then she signed them with the name the American dress-buying public had been reading about with such fascination and undisguised curiosity. She wisely kept her costs to a minimum by manufacturing in Italy, and presto! The affordable, infinitely wearable designed dress. Instead of drooling over Yves St. Laurent at $4,000 you could *have* a Diane Von Furstenberg for $70. That is, if you were into signature clothes, and in the late Sixties just about all of us were. It was like hitching your wagon to a star. Maybe if you wore a dress signed by a real-life princess you might meet a prince at the dry cleaners and live happily ever after.

In retrospect, it really doesn't matter how it began. What matters is where it went. And it went into eight figures. The suitcase full of disheveled samples, pulled out one by one at the Davenport Hotel for buyers during Market Week in 1968 (that's the version we believe)—just the samples and the instinct and a few bucks alchemized into a fifty-million-dollar empire. Behind it all is this remarkable woman, little Diane Halfin who came from a modest home in Brussels to a twelve-room Fifth Avenue co-op via the Austrian duchy of Furstenberg. Her now-familiar face and name decorate the hangtags of seventeen (at last count) separate franchises producing and selling clothing, shoes, handbags, furs, lingerie, luggage, sunglasses, jewelry and home furnishings, and are the trademark of her own cosmetics company. Along the way she had two children, Egon Alexander and Tatiana (for whom her perfume line is named), divorced her Prince, discarded her title, and dispelled for all time the notion that she couldn't cut it alone. She is one of the wealthiest and most-talked-about women of our time as well as one of its great beauties. The little girl from Brussels is not only a vast corporation, she is a household word.

She's also busy. So busy, in fact, that we had to wait months for an interview. You can imagine how pleased we were when Diane agreed to see us for an hour in New York and share her beauty ideas with us. Of all the women we met, she was the only one with her own book on the subject and most organized about not only her own beauty routines, but the role these practices can play in the lives of other women.

It was an exciting interview. For starters, the woman who now refuses to be called a princess sure lives like one. She hangs her hat in an elegant apartment high above Fifth Avenue with a panoramic view of Central Park and the reservoir. The building is in the dignified Eighties—New York's silk stocking district—and it's New York at its luxurious best. A bevvy of doormen and concierges in custom-fitted uniforms. One apartment to a floor. Very privée. Very deluxe.

We are whisked silently up to her floor by a real elevator operator (no self-service here) and greeted at her door by an Oriental butler. The trade papers once described this apartment as "operatic." Very appropriate. We walk across the needlepoint carpet, strewn with wall-to-wall roses; through the foyer with its hand-painted marble woodwork; past the dining room (upholstered in mauve and cream morning glories on chintz) with its oversized chandelier in art glass; past the living room, full of antiques and with every inch of wall space hung with art; and into the library with its cherry wood boiserie and hundreds of leatherbound books. The butler asks us to wait for her there.

Five minutes later, Diane walks brusquely into the room. The first thing you notice about her is her jewelry. She's wearing the biggest baroque pearls we've ever seen, even in the windows at Buccellati. And, along with the pearls, a heavy gold chain studded with emeralds and rubies. We try very hard not to stare; we look her in the eyes and say hello.

The familiar, somewhat feline face is bare of makeup and her dark, soft hair is loose and naturally curled. There is a casualness about her, an almost masculine disregard for her appearance. She moves as if she were in a dressing gown even though she is wearing severely tailored brown leather pants and a pink silk shirt, open nearly to her waist.

"Hello. About how long do you think this will take?" She plops on the sofa and swings her tooled leather boots up onto the cocktail table. The effect is startling. The riveting dark eyes focus in on us and, without another word, we understand that we are to begin.

It's not that she's unfriendly. She's just busy. And organized.

"When did you start to wear makeup?"

"It was very late. My God, I must have been sixteen or seventeen. I wasn't allowed to wear it at home. I was already in school in England then and I had a boyfriend who was taking me to the airport to meet my mother. She was coming to visit me at school, you see. I didn't know how to handle this situation because my mother had never seen me with makeup and my boyfriend had never seen me without, so I solved it all by saying that I had an allergy and by wearing dark glasses all day."

Even then she was fast on her feet.

And so it begins. Question. Answer. Question. Answer. Some of her responses have the ring of twice-told tales. Later we discover that she never deviates—hardly an adjective changes from her book. It might cause you to suspect that she is too well rehearsed, but our ultimate conclusion is that Diane's beauty life and beauty philosophy, like the rest of her, have found a winning direction and she sticks with it.

When she gets away from the essential facts and on to more personal material, her staggering independence and intense need for freedom come through clearly. She wrote the book, not only on DVF's beauty, but on DVF's very personal sense of liberation.

"I will never be a slave to this life I created. I built this business with my own hands but it will never own me. The most important thing for me is my freedom. I have responsibilities and people who depend on me but I have to know that I am my own person and that I control my own life. Me and nobody else, you understand? At one time I had two hundred people working for me in the United States alone. Then there was the factory in Italy. And, of course, my children, and my mother and the several friends who live with me here from time to time. Everyone I saw from the moment I awoke in the morning was dependent upon me. But it was that way because *I* wanted it that way. Having all those people needing me gave me strength, gave me my security. Without those responsibilities, I would be lost and without purpose."

It's difficult to imagine a woman with her intense look of determination being without purpose for long. Or, for that matter, ever being insecure. "Insecure? Security is very important to me. To be self-sufficient, to need to depend on no one. But personally, emotionally secure? Well, I'm not saying I'm totally sure of myself. I am like everyone else in this—I have my insecurities." She doesn't, however, mention any.

"But I don't have any insecurity about my being able to lead my own life and handle the lives of those other people. If I did, I wouldn't be here. I never wake up in the morning and say, all of this depends on me and it's too much. If it weren't for me, none of this would be here." She gestures with a sweep of her hand. It's an all-encompassing sweep and it includes us. It's a bit unnerving.

"I am, after all, very much a woman of the times. If you can communicate this and nothing else about me, it is enough. I am totally free from the old ideas about dependency and being the weaker sex. For a long time no one thought I had an identity of my own away from Egon. They wouldn't take me seriously. You see, in many ways, being the Princess Von Furstenberg made it much harder for me than for other people. They would laugh and say, what's a princess doing making dresses—and selling! My God! How could I do that! I should be dancing. Or sitting on cushions. Not out there selling a line. But you see how wrong they were. I am doing just what I should be doing. Just what I want to do. I have always been my own person. I have perseverance, good health and a belief in myself. And no one can say anything about me that I have not already said myself. I am not vulnerable because I am honest. And I am successful because I never doubted my success."

She flashes that famous sloe-eyed gaze at us, raising her lean body slightly from its semi-reclining position. "You know, doing nothing is just as difficult as doing something. So

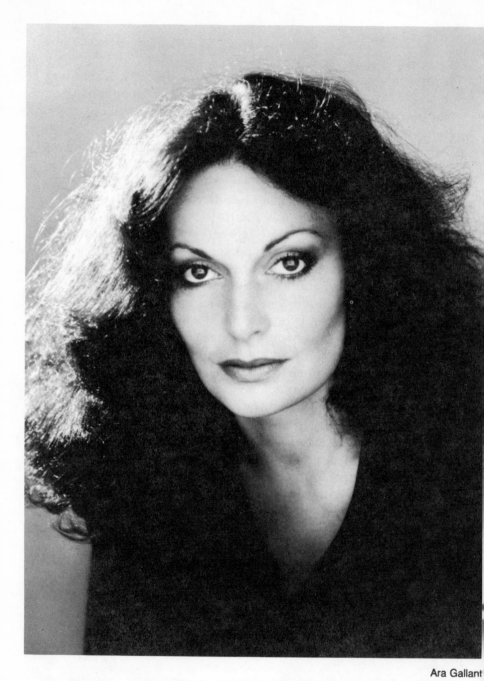

Ara Gallant

"You know, doing nothing is just as difficult as doing something. So you might as well direct your energy and your life to doing something great!"

you might as well direct your energy and your life to doing something *great!*"

Diane offers to show us her dressing room and bedroom. To get there we have to cross a carpet boundary line, going from the roses to wall-to-wall leopard skin. From the public and into the private. Her children have joined us and Tatiana is running ahead in anticipation of our reaction. Reaction to what? To the bed. You must have read somewhere about her bed. It's a $12,000 signed Dakota Jackson piece, upholstered to resemble the inside of a seashell in soft, sensuous pastel sateens. Did the artist intentionally design it to suggest Botticelli's "Venus"? That's what immediately comes to mind. The headboard is backlit so it looks as if the sun were rising up from behind. Tatiana raises and lowers the intensity of the light from a bedside control to give us the full effect. Egon Alexander strokes the coverlet. "This is where my mother sleeps," he whispers reverentially. We are impressed. Tatiana seems pleased at that and beams at us from her position at the foot of this masterpiece of light and fabric. It's a bed fit for a Capricorn. A bed fit for a princess if not for a queen.

"I was born on New Year's Eve. My birthday has always been very significant for me. When the year is over, it's really over. There can be no looking back, no rationalizing that there is still time to change the outcome. It's finished when the clock strikes twelve. When I feel oppressed by things or am too deep in the drama of my everyday life, I say to myself, how many other women have had the chances I have had, have experienced all that I have experienced. I have lived for thirty-one years—some good and some bad. But after all the pressures and the bad·things, I have come out a much stronger person, a better person—and I have developed deep understanding of life. It is worth all the effort. You only have so many cards dealt to you in this life. The trick is to play them very well."

The children are fingering her address book, gently shuffling her papers around. She asks them to leave. We go to the closet for our coats and the whole thing winds down. Diane is off giving orders to the butler and seems to have forgotten that we are still standing at the door waiting to say goodbye and thank you. The interview is over, just as abruptly as it began. There's no need to say thank you. She's moved on to other things. She's far too busy to care.

As the elevator slides up to meet us, she steps into the hallway. "Thank you," we say. "It is fine. Yes," she answers. Tatiana stands behind her, looking up.

It was, as we said, very interesting. But also a little sad. We were left with one distinct impression of the frantic and tumultuous life of this enormously successful woman. Something she said while discussing all those people gathered around her, depending on her. We asked if she ever felt the need to be alone.

"Alone?" she repeated. "Well, we are all always alone."

MAKEUP:
Diane Von Furstenberg

DIANE VON FURSTENBERG used to put her makeup on while sitting on a sink. It's still the best way she knows to get close to the mirror and that, she says, makes all the difference.

Diane thinks makeup is getting very exciting again. She should know. If anyone has her finger on the pulse of the beauty business, it's Diane. Talking with her about her makeup routine is like having a professional consultation. You can really learn from her. She's full of ideas and opinions, colors and trends. Of course she uses all of her own products. (When we suggested, half in jest, that she might have some old favorite she preferred manufactured by somebody else, she looked us straight in the eyes and said, "But why would I make it if I wouldn't use it all myself?" Touché.) So it's safe to assume that any product she describes can be purchased at the DVF cosmetics counter.

Step by step:

1. The mirror trick. Never use a magnifying mirror for makeup. It distorts the features and the balance. Get a good makeup mirror, well-lit (that's crucial) and big enough to show the entire face at once. Try to have it of a size or position where you can work close without standing.

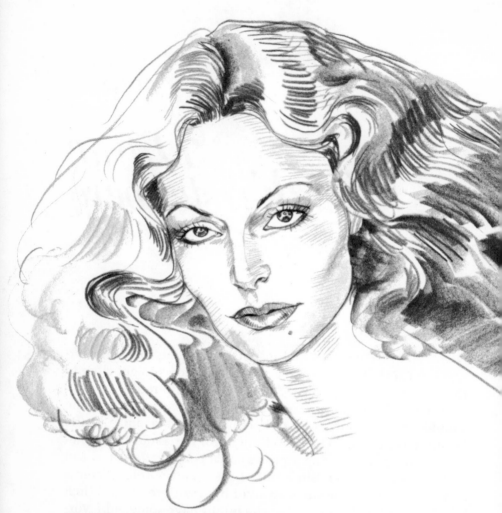

DIANE VON FURSTENBERG

THE BASE: *Pale, sheer, water-base foundation applied over moisturizer. Shading cream contouring to emphasize cheekbones. Cream blush for color on top of bone and·out to hairline. Powder blush over that, and on chin and forehead. Dusting of translucent powder.*

THE EYES: *Dramatic shadows created by paler base color and deep shadow color in crease. Highlight on brow bone. Brushed brows. Eye pencil inside lower lid to accent eye shape. Two coats of black mascara.*

THE MOUTH: *Outlined with pencil, filled in with color and gloss.*

THE FINISHED LOOK: *Extremely strong planes and dramatic eyes. Very sultry and sensual but in a softer, pinker color range now.*

2. The base. Diane cleanses with a freshening lotion and then moisturizes her face and neck. Then she applies a very light, very sheer water-base foundation. Even though she keeps an impressive array of Oriental brushes and sponges on her dressing table, she claims that the fingers are the best tool you have. The base goes on with the tips of the fingers and is blended out into nothing at the sides of the face. The skin should show through the base. The most important thing is to keep each step as sheer as possible so you can *build* (she uses this word over and over) the face without obscuring the transparency of the natural skin. It can take much longer to look natural than to look made-up but the final results are worth the extra time and effort.

3. The shading. Diane is recognized by her distinctively high cheekbones. They don't look that way by accident. She adds to their height and prominence with brown shading cream, applied directly under the bones and widened to a triangle at the hairline. She admits that she has gorgeous bones but, she adds, everyone has them—it's only necessary to find them and spiff them up a little! She works like a sculptor with the cream, blending carefully, modeling the face shape.

4. The cheek color. Next she applies a cream in any one of a number of shades from pink to red to amber. She is excited about pinks these days and is avoiding browns because she feels they are passé. The neutral face is finished. Paler, prettier and pink is in. The cheek color goes on the crest of the bone and is pulled out to the hairline and blended into the shading cream. It is important to bring the color up and out to the hairline in order to emphasize the cheekbone *and* frame and enhance the eyes.

5. The powders. Diane puts a little translucent face powder on a brush and dusts it over the face. Then she applies powdered blusher in the same (or a compatible) shade of the cream blush, once more over the top of the cheekbone and out to the hairline, lightly over the chin, and to balance, across the temples. Another light dusting of face powder over the entire face sets the base.

Now, advises Diane, sit back and take a good look at yourself. The you before your mouth and eyes are made up. It should tell you a great deal about how much or how little to emphasize these most important features. Before you begin, have a good idea just where you're heading. In any case, the balance between eyes and mouth should be carefully maintained so that the one element never overpowers the other. Your face is, at this point, a bare canvas, waiting for the focal points to be painted in.

6. The mouth. Diane is suddenly wild about pink! She never thought of herself wearing pink lipstick but it looks very right to her now—young and fresh and feminine. No matter what color direction she goes in, first she pencils the lips with a compatible color, correcting any irregularities as she goes. Then she fills in with lipstick, applied with a brush, and finishes with a touch of clear gloss.

7. The eyes. When you think about Diane Von Furstenberg, the first thing you see in your mind's eye are her deepset and glamorous eyes. Here's how she does it . . .

Always consider eye shadow as shadow, not makeup. In this way you can create dramatic eyes without looking overdone. First, select a base color, something soft and neutral like buff or beige or grey. Powder the entire lid, starting at the lashes and working up to the brow. Now select another color, a shadow color, purple or deep green or a mahogany brown. Apply this deeper tone at the crease, blending it softly into the base shadow. Then put a few dots of highlight powder just under the browline and blend. Brush your brows into shape. Diane uses an eye pencil inside the lower lid to emphasize the almond shape of her eyes and mascaras once, lets it dry, then mascaras a second time.

How long do you suppose all of this takes? Seven minutes. That's all! She's really got it down pat. But she says that with practice nearly anybody can manage an entire face in this short time and that any more is unnecessary. We're still practicing.

Here are some additional Von Furstenberg tips to keep in mind:

Try to wait at least an hour in the morning before applying makeup, to allow your face time to "sink in." Everyone's morning face is slightly swollen from sleep and it can throw off the understanding of your bones and leave you with a mess. Diane tries to stall until lunch and then does the works.

Remember to build your makeup carefully. It should never get too opaque. When you start small, you can add a little at a time all day and still look terrific. For hectic evenings, carefully intensify the colors over your morning base, and you're all set for soft lights and romance. You can start from scratch after a long day, but be sure you have enough time to cleanse thoroughly before beginning again.

Please, please be careful with shading creams! Actually, Diane feels that most of us should stay clear of them. In less than expert hands, contour creams can become deadly weapons and turn pretty, naturally soft faces into masks. It's better to let the clear skin come through and forget your slightly wandering nose or less-than-perfect chin. In any case, always remember to blend, blend, blend. The cardinal sin is a makeup line at the chin.

Never feel that it's necessary to match your makeup to your dress. A royal blue dress never made royal blue eyes pretty. If you should feel like using a little blue, by all means use a little on your eyes and then go ahead and put it on your body, but it's not necessary to coordinate the two. What's most important is to look your most beautiful—that, according to Diane, goes for makeup and for clothes. And always make the most of your best features. They can surprise you. Your best feature may be the nose you hate. It's such an important part of your personality. Don't spend hours trying to shade it into nothingness and don't, unless it's driving you to drink, search the yellow pages for a surgeon. Accept yourself. It is the biggest favor you can do for you. Diane says you might spend years never leaving the house without your makeup, then one day you do and discover that you're the very same person without your lipstick. You might even look better.

Diane Von Furstenberg at thirty-one says she's delighted to have reached a point where she has so much to offer as a mature person that she can be appealing and comfortable with or without her mascara.

Fashion

Who said:

"I resent the fact that I work so hard to stay thin and then can't wear clothes that show that I'm thin! I don't care what the fashion is, I'm going to wear things that show off my figure."

"I have hyperactive charge cards. I go into a store to buy a pair of stockings, and end up buying the world."

"Having a million dollars would mean I could buy all the clothes I want. (Does that sound awful?)"

"Last night we had friends in for dinner. I changed my clothes ten times before I settled on what I wanted to wear."

"I just buy an extra set of everything for the road."

"I can put really weird things together and they look like they were designed by someone great!"

"I love jewelry and furs. But not if I have to live on canned soup and hot dogs to buy them. You can't eat a diamond earring!"

"I absolutely refuse to pay $3,000 for a dress."

Who owns:

At least eighty-five pairs of shoes?

A sterling silver American Indian boot bracelet?

Clothes in closets in three cities?

Forty-five cashmere sweaters?

A closet for her necklaces?

An inside-out mink cape?

Flesh-colored, knee-length "nighties" in nylon chiffon?

The same style gloves in every color?

Antique belts?

The same style pants in every color?

Crazy earrings?

Unworn designer originals?

Safari suits from Africa?

At least one of everything!

Phyllis George, Suzanne Somers and Mary Tyler Moore all had one thing in common. Jeans. Marisa, Cheryl, Diane and Jackie all wore jeans, too, but Marisa's were Fiorucci green-jeans, Cheryl's came with studs and a script in the pocket, Diane's were leather, worn with no underwear, and Jackie's were delicious suede. Jackie's also happened to be the identi-cal pair she wears in *Someone Is Killing the Great Chefs of Europe.*

Wardrobe Come Home seems to be a popular second feature and fringe benefit among the stars!

Olivia wore fatigues—unfatigued. (They were starched and pressed.) Liv wore a leotard and gypsy skirt. Ann-Margret was demure in an apricot fur-blend dress. And Margaux wore mix-and-match outrageous.

Taken as a whole, they care—really care—about clothes. That shouldn't surprise anyone. It seems that dressing well and with strong personal style comes hand in glove with being a successful beauty. What was interesting were the frequent claims to fashion independence among them. Perhaps, when you've got so much going for you already, you can afford (both aesthetically and financially) to thumb your nose at the readily available and hot-ticket items. And the authorities like *Vogue* and *Bazaar*. In any event, even those fashion independents whose wardrobes were built around Levi-Strauss managed to make jeans look custom. For one thing, they fit like nobody's business. As if they were pinned to the form at the tailor's. Even the T-shirts were impeccable. Everything had the distinct aura of big $$$ and sported the knife-edge crease of the French dry cleaner.

Let's face it. There are no happy hands at home in the upper echelons. These people definitely don't compare laundry detergents over a light lunch, or use Spray and Wash on the tattletale grey. It is refreshing to note, however, that their attitude toward what they wear shows a definite tendency away from the "clothes make the man" philosophy and a trend to a more sensible, down-to-earth approach we all can adopt. Basically, they all agreed that the dress should never wear the woman. And no one would quarrel with that advice!

Take Mary Tyler Moore, for example. Mary said right off that she's not a clothes horse. At the time, she was standing there in a pair of perfectly cut and fitted blue jeans and a lipstick-red cotton T-shirt. Her only nod to coordination were the navy canvas espadrilles on her feet. She's kept the same simple, uncluttered, tailored look (with minor changes of length and detailing) first designed for her by Norman Todd in 1970. To Mary, a jazzy change is the addition of a silk scarf and some gold chains. The day we met her, the first thing we noticed was her smile. And you'd better believe that wasn't an accident. Under the cotton-knit skin of this understated dresser there beats the heart of a very savvy woman. Mary's simple cotton skirts and coordinating shirts, or jeans and tees, never compete with Mary the *person*. They flatter her, complement her low-key and likable image. But her clothes never make an entrance before she does.

She will not, for example, wear fur. She doesn't believe in it. Not because it's extravagant, but because she loves animals. And—this knocked us right off our feet—she is anti oversized blousy silhouettes, *not* because she is petite and could be swallowed alive by a Kenzo bigtop but because, as she succinctly put it, she works too hard to keep that figure to hide it away under ten yards of cotton lawn. She'll choose jersey every time. Clingers. And a touch of décolleté. Not too much. But never too little. Mary also loves lacy underthings. Little floaty "nighties" in chiffon. Nude colored. What a surprising woman she is! Just a hint of a tease.

Cheryl Ladd's only fashion comment during our hectic hour together was that she too loves lacy lingerie and, from time to time, will slip into a satin nightgown and her favorite perfume as an alternative to an after-dinner drink for David. Prosit!

Jackie Bisset travels with a big, black trunk. In it, surrounded by tissue and hung on individual hangers, is nearly everything she owns. When Jackie takes a trip, she takes everything but the kitchen sink. This, she claims, is due to lack of time for her packing as much as indecisiveness. It's easier to take more. But Jackie is not, *definitely* not, the sort who depends on her wardrobe to get her through. She enjoys clothes but she enjoys people more.

Jackie told us an interesting anecdote about a fancy party she had attended a few evenings before. A beautiful woman, not young, not old, had arrived in a gorgeous ensemble, replete with turban and chiffon scarves. She stood, moved, posed through the evening—perfectly pulled together but not speaking or relating to the other guests. She seemingly needed only to be there to let her clothes do all her talking. Jackie found her fascinating. Here was someone who either was hiding her insecurities in a thousand-dollar dress or else had her priorities all wrong. No one was impressed. They just avoided her. "What a pity," said La Bisset. "She might have been an interesting person. But no one could get through all that chiffon to reach her. That little extravaganza turned into an isolation booth in high-heeled slippers."

You can always get past the outfit and on to Jackie Bisset. She has an ability to toss anything she puts on right into the shadow of Jackie the *woman*. Even furs and jewelry. She's got a wonderful collection of funny little rings, old ones and new ones all mixed up together. And she loves crazy earrings. But her earrings never lead you away from her eyes and the rings take second place to her expressive hands. Then there's the story of that incredible mink cape Vic (her man of the moment) gave her. She's not sure whether or not she's wearing it the right way. Her own sense of style, and sense of humor, gave this unlined fur a new twist—a 180-degree twist to be exact. She wears the thing inside out. Only Jackie could carry it off.

Olivia Newton-John has travel trauma. Touring around as she does, she hits several climates in the course of one sing and fly. This means seasonal changes of wardrobe, like packing for a trip to Alaska, Houston and Rio de Janeiro. Olivia solves it by taking one of everything. Traveling this way can become complicated, she admits. Particularly when you love clothes as much as she does and, therefore, own almost more than you can ever wear. At least during a three-week tour. What makes matters worse is that she inevitably picks up a few things wherever she works, like the safari suits she brought home from her ABC filming in Africa. But when it comes to basic accessories and makeup, she's given up completely. Rather than trying to remember everything, she buys an extra set for the road. Now she never forgets her favorite shoes or her favorite lipstick.

What lingers in our minds about Olivia's fashion presence, however, is the color she wore. Khaki. Khaki trousers, cut in the relaxed style of Marine fatigues. And the most beautiful khaki wool sweater. Her natural leather boots and cream silk shirt finished it off on such a low color key that on anyone save Olivia (with her brilliant blue eyes and sunlit hair) the whole effect might have been *blah.* How wonderful she looked that day! As she raced around between cuts at the recording studio, her clothes remained at-ease. Nothing overstated, nothing competitive. Infinitely flattering to her natural good looks.

It was Friday, and Marisa was flamboyant. Red light! Green light! Nothing low-key or timid about Berenson. Her colors popped like flashbulbs. She's had the most practice, of course. She was dressed by the pros during her modeling years, aiding and abetting their knowhow with her own spectacular instincts. And on that Friday afternoon she carried off an outfit that might have eaten the less confident for lunch. Screaming green. Skinny, skinny Fiorucci jeans and a tiny little tee to match. And those funny red patent oxfords! The sort of shoe you might buy on impulse, then never have the guts to wear. The granddaughter of Mme. Schiaparelli, however, never bats an eye when it comes to pulling herself together. In the front lines every time. It is always Marisa wearing *le dernier cri* and never the other way around. Brave soul. She will bare it, layer it, blouse it, skinny it down, whatever her freethinking, freewheeling fashion sense senses is new. Cover herself with fur and jewels. Drape herself in yards of chiffon. Spin down a staircase into a crowded room. Marisa Berenson is far more than fashionable. She *is* fashion.

Having this intense love for clothes has its problems. Marisa, who has several residences spread across the globe, says she is always packing. Not your basic weekender, by any means. Scores of matched pieces. An army of Louis Vuitton. And, inevitably, just the perfect thing always ends up, not in the attic, but in Paris—when she's in L.A. Or vice versa. Or, worse yet, lost in the maw of her endless closets. In fact, when Marisa was pregnant, she was spared that frustrating ritual of shopping maternity departments where everything is designed to turn the expectant mother into the Hindenburg. She just pried open some long-ago and far-away closets in Paris and discovered a cache of gorgeous, full, figure-concealing dresses and tops she had purchased in the long-distant past. If you love clothes, just the thought can take your breath away. Miles and miles of hangers. Continents of hatboxes. Shoes stretching to the vanishing point. If she ever holds a garage sale, we'll be the first in line.

Getting back down to earth, there's Liv Ullmann. Liv is a warm and lovely lady. She kept complimenting *us* on our choice of dress. She feels she has no talent whatever in this area. We suspect that she has never had a driving emotional need to learn, concerning herself as she does with her tremendous acting talent and her family and friends. Talking face to face with Liv, you could never imagine her dressed to the nines and out partying, night after night. She is a very basic woman of great depth and her choice of clothing reflects this.

Designers and well-meaning friends have tried to "coordinate" her. Some have even designed especially for her and sent over expensive, beautiful garments or mini wardrobes. They come in, are hung on hangers, and there they stay. She may try them on and admire the workmanship or the color or the print. But she rarely wears them. All that is not for her. Liv does own some fine jewelry, but she rarely wears it. "Coming from a part of the world where the politics and the thinking are traditionally socialistic, I can't find it in my heart to wear flashy jewels when all around me people don't have enough to eat. It would make me feel guilty. You understand?" We understand.

Diane Von Furstenberg, on the other hand, wore pearls. Baroque pearls so big they could send a kid through college. And a Bulgari neck chain forged of solid gold, rubies and emeralds. We don't mean to say that Diane is self-indulgent to the exclusion of others. As she put it, "I love to take care of other people. But I choose to take care of myself first." There is a total lack of guilt in Diane. She really enjoys her life-style and all the things that hard-earned money can buy. She took us on a rapid tour of her own rooms, including her dressing room and closets. A quick glance told us that Diane Von Furstenberg doesn't wear many Diane Von Furstenbergs or, if she does, she leaves them at the office. What we saw was silk. And leather. (And, unlike cotton/fortrel, this won't wash!) She does *believe* in what she designs, but for her interview she chose a pale pink silk shirt, open nearly to the waist, and second-skin mahogany leather jeans. Unlike the little DVF dress, this look is definitely *not* flattering on everybody. It is almost unbearably sexy on Diane, who chooses to make sex appeal a big part of her style and her business. Added to the really provocative feeling of silks and skins was the tantalizing admission that she wears no underwear. And you can *tell* that she wears no underwear. Diane is *quite* a woman. Would you expect less from a person who keeps a trampoline in her rose-strewn private bath?

The bottom line on DVF on fashion is that she's a professional dresser. She works for an effect and she understands exactly what she's doing. She looks as sexy in an oversized man's shirt as she does in silk pajamas. Anyone with that level of expertise doesn't need to buy haute couture. As a young bride she covered the European collections, gathering instant-status clothes along with some pretty hefty price tags. No more. Diane doesn't need to pay $3,000 for a dress. Particularly when nothing she wears these days ever upstages Diane. An observant man friend was overheard to remark, "Diane always looks as if she's about to remove her clothes!"

Margaux Hemingway mixes and matches on the spot. She can throw together some of the most imponderable combinations and make them work. Highly individual, this girl. Months before they were being seen in New York, Margaux wore her pants just to the ankle and skinnied down from the hip. With a striped silk tux shirt. And a ponytail. And high-heeled pumps. She really likes the *people* who design the clothes, admires their creativity and spirit and thinks they're fun. Especially Halston. And some of the above must have rubbed off on Margaux. She manages to assemble some pretty weird pieces and look straight off the runway! All on her own.

Phyllis George, Ann-Margret and Suzanne Somers are the heavies in this piece. The all-out clothes freaks. Phyllis, who tried to fool us by arriving in blue jeans and a T-shirt, has a real problem with her charge cards. Her Bloomingdale's account, for example, changes figures faster than the Dow Jones Index. She can go into a store on an innocent errand for a pair of stockings and exit with at least one of everything. If she happens to find a perfect pair of gloves that come in ten delicious shades: One of each, please, size seven, sign right here. Or the perfect pant. Oh, they come in five colors and two plaids? One of each, please. And she leaves her autograph in Better Sportswear.

This method cuts down on shopping time and helps her coordinate for a trip which, in the "commentating" business, can involve a lot of climates and lots of changes. Phyl is a "freak" for blazers. And vests. And tailored things. She has a bag to go with everything. And oodles of boots. And scarves. And on. And on. She claims to be the world's greatest shopper. Give her two hours and she can buy the *world*. You have to smile as she talks about it. Her love of clothing is so out front and shameless. "Feeling well-dressed makes me feel good inside," says the girl who'll top off her Maverick jeans with a $200 Yves St. Laurent shirt without batting an eye. "Why Yves St. Laurent? Or Valentino? Extravagant, maybe. But every time I put it on I feel like a million dollars! That's why."

Phyl *doesn't* like sexy clothes. At least not blatantly sexy clothes. She doesn't mind a little cleavage, but when the neckline falls to the navel that's too far. Suzanne Somers agrees. Suzanne, who, as Chrissy, elevated the towel to the Coty Award Hall of Fame, doesn't really believe in suggestive clothing. It makes other people uncomfortable. A little bareness, a clinging yard of jersey or two, that's just fine. But Suzanne has a foolproof way of checking her costumes before she sets foot out of the dressing room. She imagines that she will be at dinner with two men and their wives. If the husbands would be hard pressed to tear their eyes away from whatever part of her anatomy is straining at the seams, she's gone too far. And off it comes. A more demure number goes to dinner. "If you can be appealing without being threatening, then you've got the perfect, feminine look."

Suzanne would rather shop than eat. But not if shopping for clothes meant living on hot dogs the rest of the month. She's a pragmatist about luxuries, having done without for so many years. She once had a diamond engagement ring, a leftover from her first marriage, and nothing to eat. "You'd be surprised how little those things can mean, even if you love pretty jewelry, when you're hungry. I sold that ring to the first jeweler I could find. Not a moment's hesitation. Now, after the rent's been paid, the refrigerator stocked, and a little bundle's been socked away, maybe an extravagance. Never before."

Even though she buys quantities of clothes, Suzanne shops wisely. Years of meager-budget buying taught her to choose quality over quantity, classics over fads. "Even as a child, I would have one special outfit a season, maybe a cashmere sweater and a good skirt and jacket. No matter how many times I wore it, I always knew I looked put together. It was a sure thing. I wore uniforms to school as a girl, so that one outfit was all I needed. It was a terrific lesson to learn."

Things have changed a bit for Suzanne. But she still *loves* bargains and there's a twinkle of girlish delight in her voice when she admits that having a million dollars would mean she could buy all the clothes she could ever want. Then she ducks her head a little, looks up in penitent innocence and adds, "Does that sound *awful?*" Frankly, coming from her, it sounds like fun.

Last, but far from least, we have Ann-Margret's closet. We could do an hour-long special on Ann-Margret's closet. First of all it's bigger than an average master bedroom. About twelve feet by eighteen feet. And it's totally cedar lined. The smell in that closet is as sweet as a forest. It's fitted with endless drawers, shoe cubbies and hat stands. And *full.* Full to overflowing. At least one of everything you can think of, and multiples of many things. Scores of cashmere sweaters are neatly rolled and coddled in tissue in drawers. Dozens of chapeaux march around the top shelves. Handbags are stacked to the ceiling. Somewhere just under 100 pairs of shoes and boots fill up the pigeonholes on one long wall. Along another wall there are racks. Hundreds of skirts, dresses, shirts and pants hang there, all arranged by color and season. Something old, something new, something yellow, something blue. Something black. She reaches for it and pulls it out. It's a black silk smock from Yves St. Laurent, advertised in last month's *Vogue* for $595. She doesn't mention the cost, but holds it out with the ingenuous excitement of a child and we understand that the cost doesn't matter.

There's more. The adjacent dressing room has an unusual kind of wainscotting which, on closer inspection, turns out to be closet doors. Designed by her husband, Roger (as was all of this organization), these closets are home to her accessories. Costume jewelry. Gloves. Scarves. Belts. Skinny drawers for earrings. Medium-sized drawers for bracelets. Pullout racks with hooks for belts. More doors swing open. Here are velvet display boards with hooks for necklaces, pendants, pearls and gold chains. You've got to know the system in here. Memorize exact locations. Pink pearl earrings, clipback, with gold leaves, drawer #6A, north wall, center section, third from bottom. Everything's coded and filed away. Imagine sleeping through the alarm, then stumbling in here, half asleep, and trying to find a pair of stockings or a white silk scarf? Mayhem. This system was designed for a woman with some serious time on her hands. Someone who enjoys browsing around for the perfect finishing touch. Definitely not a nine-to-fiver. She is standing there, in the middle of her own private Saks Fifth Avenue, beaming with delight. What a picture she draws when she tells us how she changed her clothes ten times the other night before deciding on the perfect hostess ensemble in which to welcome her dinner guests. In her ripe apricot furry dress with its drawstring tie and her nude-colored sandals, she bends and reaches, opening drawer after drawer, cabinet after cabinet until we are hypnotized and speechless with the wonder of it all.

Almost without exception, they complimented us. "What a

terrific dress!" "I love your shawl!" Made us feel special and important and, in some cases, contributory. Like one of the girls, sharing sales and copping secrets. So we told them where to go for this or that in New York. Or smiled and graciously accepted their praise on our choice of shoes or jacket. And, in the end, this was what stuck in our minds. How open they were and how interested—these women with their nearly infinite resources and wardrobe ladies and highly personal styles. After all, who better than they understands what part fashion should play in the overall picture. These women who can step into a movie theater and watch themselves walk across a room. Or who have five hundred critics in the audience every night. Or millions watching on the tube. Or who design or model fashion for billions all over the world. Few of us, if any, will ever have the advantages of these eleven—the expert guidance and constant critical appraisal to which they have access every day of their working lives. Yet *they* asked *us*. Where did we buy the skirt? Well, we confessed. So if you're ever at Loehmann's in the Bronx, reaching for a $100 sweater marked $29.95, the blonde holding the other sleeve might just be Suzanne.

P.S. If you're still in the dark about who the who said and the who owns, here are the answers:

Who said:
1. Mary Tyler Moore
2. Phyllis George
3. Suzanne Somers
4. Ann-Margret
5. Olivia Newton-John
6. Margaux Hemingway
7. Suzanne Somers
8. Diane Von Furstenberg

Who owns:
1. Ann-Margret
2. Jacqueline Bisset
3. Marisa Berenson
4. Ann-Margret
5. Ann-Margret
6. Jacqueline Bisset
7. Mary Tyler Moore
8. Phyllis George
9. Suzanne Somers
10. Phyllis George
11. Jacqueline Bisset
12. Liv Ullmann
13. Olivia Newton-John
14. Ann-Margret

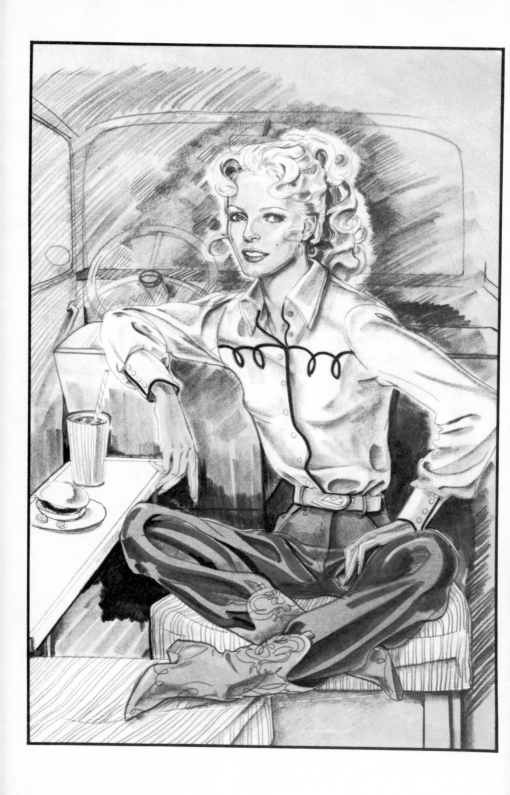

Cheryl Ladd

THE SIGN on the door says DO NOT ENTER WHEN THE RED LIGHT IS FLASHING!

Blip. Blip. Blip. But the blonde with the ponytail and the size-four jeans tosses her head as a signal for us to follow and barges right in.

We've never seen anything like it. The sound stage is as big as a convention hall and twice as high. Miles of cables swing from catwalks and dangle from the overhead equipment. We clatter across the concrete floor, past the Mr. Coffee and the table of half-eaten breakfast rolls, following that twitching ponytail, moving toward a far corner of the huge stage where the artificial daylight hangs in the hot air like a halo. We round a twelve-foot stage flat.

"Ssssshhhhhhhh! Keep it *down* over there! This is a take!" We stop dead in our tracks. We've walked smack into the filming of *Charlie's Angels*.

There is something very funny about the set. You see, you just can't get a grip on what you're looking at. In front of you is a garage. The real thing—old cars with dents, an office with a cashier and all these people milling around looking like they've lost their claim checks. But beyond the corolla of the

175

klieg lights are all these *other* people. Hunched over. Whispering. Sounding very important or very hassled, shouting orders. Answering in cadence. "Sound!" "Speed!" "Camera one, ready?" "Ready on one!"

"Okay, okay. Scene ten. Take four. Places!" "Places, everybody!"

Who is the director? Who can tell! Who is real, who is acting? The crew scurries around and then settles into position. There's a grey-haired man on a big mobile camera with its own chair right beside us. He sounds disgusted. "Ready on camera two." Another voice. "Got a reading, camera two?" "Lights?" "We're hot." More mumbo jumbo. Everyone looks busy. We scrunch ourselves up against a wall and try to disappear.

"Okay, Cheryl. From your entrance."

A little bit of a girl walks from the pseudo-office into the brilliant glare of the set lights. Her hair is white-blond and blinding bright. She is tiny, tiny. No bigger than 5'4", probably no heavier than a toy terrier. Her perfect features are set in a businesslike deadpan as she steps into character. She's wearing black jeans, so excruciatingly tight we hope there will be no sitting scenes, and a black and white cowgirl shirt. It's then that we notice that it's the exact outfit our ponytailed girl guide is wearing. Except for the hairdo, they're a matched set. Cheryl's stand-in takes our lunch orders as the scene begins.

Have you ever wondered if the man with the black and white striped chalkboard really jumps out in front of the camera and says, *"Charlie's Angels,"* episode number 157, scene ten, take four!" and then clicks that clicker board together? He does. Except that by now it is "Scene ten, take five." (Due to some technical error.) The director yells "Action" and everyone suddenly starts moving. Out comes a disheveled (and obviously suspect) antihero-type character actor with a paper cup of coffee. He lurches into the garage set and starts to fumble with the door of a '69 Chevvy when, right on cue, carrying a little cops and robbers clipboard comes Cheryl—all dolled up and alluringly investigative and so damn pretty you figure that the suspect antihero will confess if only she'll have dinner with him tonight.

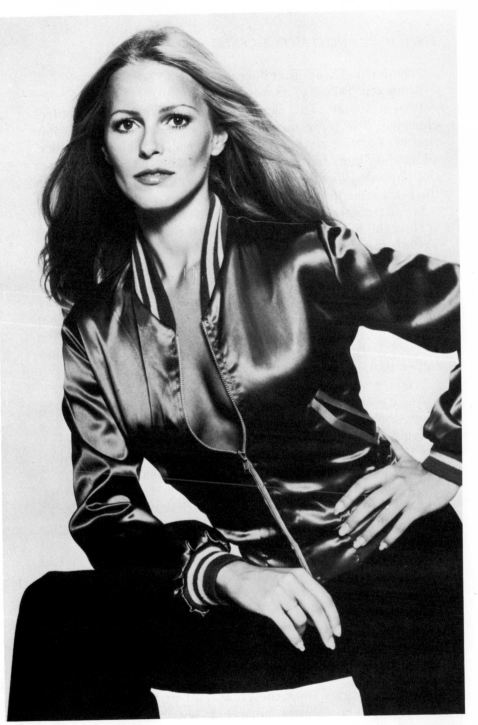

Harry Langdon

Wonderful. Except that the car door didn't open.

Scene ten. Take six.

Instant replay. The same Houston Space Center Control checklist. The same movements, the same words, the same timing. For the sixth time, Cheryl walks out of the office, swings her body to the right at the marker on the floor, passes the clipboard to the cop behind her and says "Hi, there!" in the exact same tone of voice. Whoops!

Scene ten, take seven. (Antihero blew his lines.)

Now the hairdresser comes out of the darkness armed with a comb and some blond bobby pins. Cheryl's hair is looking a bit less than stunning. She is also a bit less than ready.

Scene ten, take eight. (Cheryl blew her lines.)

We're having a wonderful time by now. Really in the swing of things. Very familiar with the dialogue. ("I understand that you were the last person to see the victim alive?" "Yeh. She was my last fare before coming back to the garage. A lousy tipper, too!") Wait a minute! That wasn't in there before!

Scene ten, take nine.

Ah, c'mon, you guys! Get it together! We keep thinking about that cold cup of coffee the taxi driver (murderer!) is swigging, and our yogurt and fresh fruit salads waiting for us out there somewhere. Let's get it *down*! Now, not only does cameraman #2 look disgusted, everyone looks disgusted.

Take nine has an unusable beginning and an okay ending. At least no one tripped over the cables or was off the mark.

The director decides to compromise. To splice. The beginning of take four (isn't that where we came in?) and the end of take nine. (Well, that is *definitely* where we go *out*. We've had it. It is about 103 degrees in here and if we have to watch it all fall apart one more time we'll scream!)

"Lunch. Let's take a break. Put scene ten in the can, Jim. Back on the set in one hour, please, ladies and gentlemen!"

Cheryl Ladd, superstar, reels out of the set, beads of perspiration on her powdered forehead, still *smiling*, politely answering questions from the crew, patiently listening to the hairdresser who advises putting a few hot curlers in her bangs. She threads her way through the equipment to where we stand waiting to be introduced to the girl we've watched at work for over an hour. We feel as if we've known her for a long, long time.

"How very nice to see you! Have you been here long? Gee, I guess we weren't at our best today. Too bad. A little tired. All of us. Have you had lunch? Let's go to the trailer where we can sit down. I've been on my feet since six and I'm *starved!*"

God, is this any way to earn a living? She looks exhausted. Beautiful, but exhausted.

The big stage door swings open and we are blinded by the sunlight. Inside it was hot, timeless, all life centering on that paper garage and what was said there. Outside, the world goes round.

Our eyes finally adjust to the daylight and we walk to the big Winnebago, following the blonde in the size-four jeans named Cheryl.

There is no star on the door. But for Cheryl Stoppelmoor, born thirty years ago in Huron, South Dakota, the star is there—as surely as if it were buffed up every morning by one of the hundreds of people who surround her these days, advising, supporting or simply cheering her on. And if ever this pint-sized package had doubts about herself and her career, you'd never guess. Cheryl is clearly on her way. And she's deliriously happy about it.

"I'm just where I always wanted to be, able to do what I've always known I can do best. Entertaining. I'm in a fabulous career situation. When I joined *Angels* the part of Chris was *the* part to land. People said, 'Cheryl Ladd? Who's she?' I had a lot to prove to everybody. But it's all worked out so well! We all get along. I feel so good about the role and about what I'm doing. And more importantly, I feel good about *me*. Here I am, little Cheryl Stoppelmoor, the girl everyone in Huron thought was crazy because she was a nobody and she wanted to be in show business from day one. I mean, almost from the time I began to talk. Here I am, in touch with all the things I ever wanted in my life. I have a wonderful, supportive, loving husband and a beautiful child. That's most important. And I

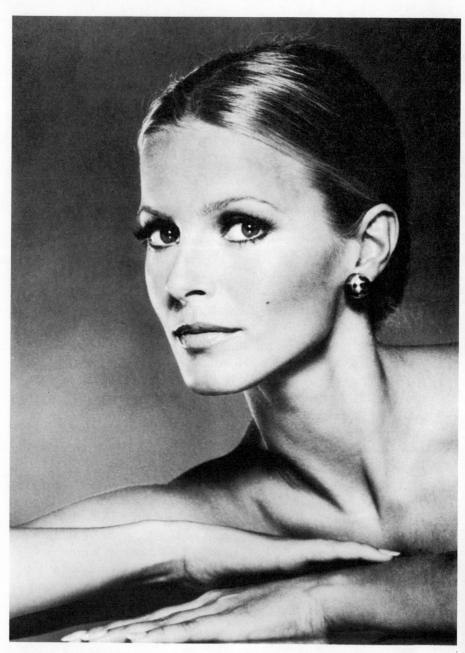

Harry Langdon

have the belief that I *am* somebody and am free to choose to be the best I can be in a business I love. Being happy about yourself without jealousy and without guilt. That's the ultimate goal in life."

She looks every inch the happy, successful young woman she's described, sitting here in her comfortable trailer gustily eating her lunch. Cheryl is as wholesome and as all-American as apple pie. She radiates unstudied honesty. She's also got her priorities in order. Her affection for her husband and her three-year-old child bubbles up in her voice:

"Jordan. Jordan Elizabeth. David and I want above all for her to have a happy life. We protect her from all the publicity as well as we can. And we try to make every minute we spend with her count. She visits me on the set a lot. Everyone here knows her and loves her. She's so aware of all that's going on that when the buzzer sounds for silence on the set, she puts her little finger up to her mouth and goes, 'SSSSShhhhh!' To her, all of this is no different than if I worked in an office. She's a very normal, unspoiled little girl. What's important is that she can see what I do when I'm working and not with her. It was a hard decision for me, to leave her and go to work on this show. We're very close, the three of us. It had to be the right choice for all of us. Since David is an actor, he understood and encouraged me to go back to work. But we worried about Jordan. Then a friend reminded us that no one has to be with a child twenty-four hours a day to be a good parent. Quality time is what counts. You can show just as much love and caring in a few hours as you can in a whole day. Now she's happy, and we're happy, and the guilt is gone for good!"

Cheryl Ladd is very likable. Her responses to our questions are honest and as fresh as her apple-cheeked good looks. All around her, on every tabletop and ledge in the Winnebago, are framed photographs of David and Jordan. There's not a single publicity still of "Cheryl the Star." There's Jordan at the beach with a pail and shovel. Jordan in the pool. David and Jordan. David alone, ruggedly handsome and laughing. It's very comfortable in here. We're beginning to feel like old friends.

Someone raps on the trailer door. "Miss Ladd. Ten minutes."

Cheryl unwinds the curlers from her hair. She sighs and pushes away the uneaten half of her lunch on its paper plate. "Seems like I never get to finish *anything* around here!"

Then she smiles and turns those baby blues on us and says, "I think the most important thing to remember about personal beauty is that it's part of the whole package. There's a Cinderella inside us all, just waiting to be discovered. But it has to do with more than a pretty face. Who you are, how much you like yourself, how you speak, what you do, how you deal with your life, how you relate to people—how you look is a small part of it. I've always admired women who are bright, well-informed and secure about themselves, even if they aren't the most beautiful in the room. What you're wearing, your hair, your makeup, your facial and bodily beauty, that's all frosting on the cake. The cake is the *person* you are."

Another discrete knock. "Miss Ladd. Time."

We file out the narrow trailer door, back into the sunlight and the beautiful Los Angeles day. To the right, the streets of *Funny Girl* sleep in the afternoon heat. Behind us, the New York Public Library lions snore away undisturbed. In front is a paper and tin Third Avenue El. All the silent ghost towns of the Twentieth Century-Fox lot are spread around us like so many attic closets. The mothball fleet. The stuff of which dreams are made.

A very real and vibrant Cheryl Stoppelmoor Ladd waves goodbye and goes back to work. We watch her stride off in the direction of the sound stage, her fatigue vanished, her natural ebullience propelling her along. Wife, working mother, and star. But most interesting of all, a very *human* being.

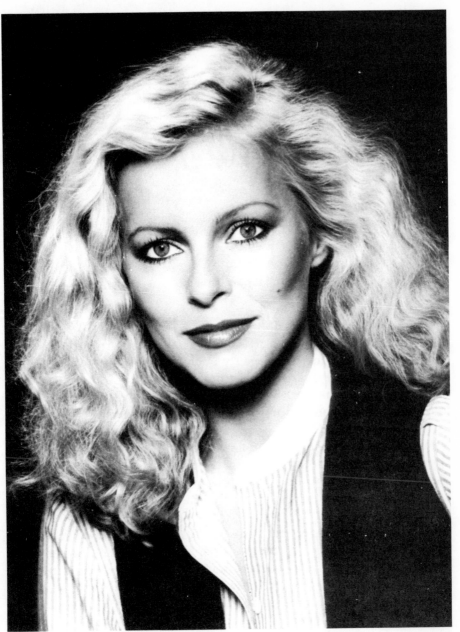

Harry Langdon

*"The most important thing to remember about personal
beauty is that it's part of the whole package. There's a
Cinderella inside us all, just waiting to be discovered."*

MAKEUP:

Cheryl Ladd

CHERYL LADD HAS perfect features. Of all the women we interviewed, hers was the real "beauty book" face. Nothing too big or too small. Not even an irregular eyelash. She's a relative newcomer to makeup, having been unable to decide as a young girl between lipstick and climbing trees (the two being incompatible at the time). In fact, Cheryl says she's only learned how to really use makeup in the last year or two, presumably because of her repeated association with professional makeup men. Even the pros would have a hard time finding a problem to correct on that face. Mother Nature has dealt her a hand full of aces.

Cheryl has problem skin, she says. You'd never know it. She uses Neutrogena and a cold water splash with an astringent chaser twice a day and she lets her skin breathe by avoiding any makeup at all on her off-the-set days. Pancake and hot lights in constant combination add to her troubles, so cleanliness is a must. Sneaking around the local playground with Jordan, barefaced with pigtails, even her lack of mascara won't allow her to go unrecognized anymore. So she acquiesces to her fame with a flick of mascara and a slick of lip gloss and goes off to the market.

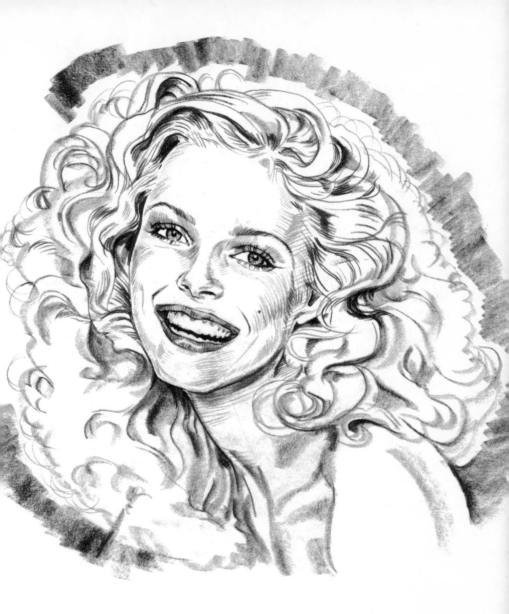

CHERYL LADD

THE BASE: *Soap and water and a cold splash, very little foundation, powdered blush in a natural shade. No contouring for normal wear.*

THE EYES: *Soft brown shadows; very little brown mascara, and brows brushed up. No pencils or liners.*

THE MOUTH: *Light lipstick pencil outline and then soft natural color, straight from the tube.*

THE FINISHED LOOK: *Very Californian, outdoor-girl and healthy. Clean, clean, clean.*

When she does wear more, subtlety is the rule. A dot or two of foundation to cover any trouble spots and a once-over with powdered blusher; lipstick straight from the tube in a soft, natural color and she's done with her skin and mouth. And her eyes? Same rules. Quiet brown powder shadows put on with a brush rather than a sponge, and a little bit of brown mascara. Then she brushes her natural brows up and she's ready. Even for the most gala evenings, Cheryl thinks that less is more.

We asked if she had any makeup tricks she could pass along. "No," she replied. "I have too many more important things in my life right now. All I can say is that if there is a part of you you *really* don't like, perhaps it's better to think of having it changed rather than spending all that time with concealing or contour creams. The most important thing is that you keep it all in perspective. Your makeup just isn't you, is it?"

$\mathcal{G}rowing\,\mathcal{O}ld$

"Who dreamed that beauty passes like a dream."
WILLIAM BUTLER YEATS

"And, as for me, I don't think I'll take it very well!"
JACQUELINE BISSET

THEY WILL GROW OLD. We all grow old. There is some comfort in the commonality of the process. But what if you're not of the common mold? If you're special, set apart, exceptionally beautiful? Faces gain character with age, grow handsome, look comfortable as worn slippers. But beauty passes. And the passage of extraordinary beauty, beauty professionally spotlit and filmed and photographed like a freeze-frame chronicle of the passing of time is a poignant and a fearful process. For them, there is so much more to lose.

"I think about growing old often. Very often. In this business it's essential to be young and beautiful. I play a girl of nineteen or twenty. Sure, I can arrange my hair, adjust my makeup—now. I'm thirty-one. But I can't do those things forever. As a private person I want to believe that beauty is merely a matter of attitude. That you can be beautiful at fifty. But as a professional, I know that it's not that simple. Sure I'd have plastic surgery if my neck started to sag and my eyes got baggy. If I can afford it, and it makes it easier for me emotionally, why not?"

SUZANNE SOMERS (31)

"You only get better! You may not look better, of course, but you get better. It's purely a matter of skin type—who ages well and who doesn't. And if you don't—have a face lift. But I would never let my face get taut and masklike from too much lifting. It's better to have some wrinkles. After all, every little wrinkle means something."

DIANE VON FURSTENBERG (31)

"I find the process of growing older an exciting experience. Of course, I was raised in Europe where there is no real emphasis on youth the way there is here. I've no fear of age. I enjoy watching my feelings about myself maturing and growing. I can play more profound parts. The loss of youthful beauty means nothing to me. No one ever told me I was beautiful as a child, so I grew up without feeling I had something so precious to lose."

ANN-MARGRET (40+)

"I'm not threatened, not at all. If I needed to, I'd have plastic surgery. My mother just had her eyes done and she looks and feels terrific. For me—so far—older has been better. I've lost all the puppy fat and my face looks much more 'settled-in' than it did when I was Miss America. I photograph better now. I guess when the time comes to deal with it, I will. I'll smile. Smiling makes you beautiful. Age can't affect the beauty of a smile!"

PHYLLIS GEORGE (30)

"Intelligence—self-awareness—security—are all important. Aging isn't important. Beauty is a much bigger thing than youth. Sure, for some of us, plastic surgery is sensible. If you look ten years older than you should because your eyes are baggy or you've wrinkled too early. It's the same as coloring your hair if you are prematurely grey. If you feel less than your best and can do something cosmetically or surgically to remedy the problem, to help your mental attitude and your self-esteem, then by all means, do it! Of course, no one should try to look twenty when they're forty. It's not natural. A lot of women are beautiful after forty."

CHERYL LADD (30)

"Being considered physically beautiful can be a liability. It's hard for people to get past that and on to your spiritual beauty. The older I get, the better I feel about myself."

MARISA BERENSON (31)

"I try not to think about it. I just want to keep the bounce in my life!"

JACQUELINE BISSET (34)

"I just can't wait to start collecting those wrinkles! It's so healthy! My grandmother has a wonderful face full of wrinkles and yet she's all energy and so in tune with herself and everything around her. I may change my mind, you know, when it starts to happen to me, but right now I feel that aging is the most natural human process and I can't wait!"

MARGAUX HEMINGWAY (24)

"First off, I don't fancy operations! Some of my friends have had plastic surgery and they feel much better about themselves afterwards. All I can say is that I hope I can age as gracefully as my mother has."

OLIVIA NEWTON-JOHN (31)

"I hate the emphasis on youth in this country! I think it's damaging. We all get older, but there is so much more to life than youth. I loved what Jane Fonda said when asked what it felt like to turn forty: 'It feels wonderful! What really hurt me was turning thirty because then youth was all I had and I hated to lose it!' But if it means a great deal to you to try to correct the physical signs of aging, by all means do it! After all, plastic surgery is really just an extension of putting on your mascara."

MARY TYLER MOORE (40+)

"I have often said that I have no fear of growing old. I don't know if that is true anymore. I have this little nagging fear that the part of me to which people respond the most strongly has to do with my sensuality, with my sexuality, rather than wih my whole person—that when I am older and less attractive sexually, I will be less attractive as a human being. Rationally, I know that this is not so, that I will remain the same human being. But the fear is still there. That I will be less wanted, less valued, when my youth has gone."

LIV ULLMANN (40+)

"That I will be less wanted, less valued, when my youth has gone." Is there anyone who hasn't felt this at one moment or another? Can you find yourself among them? To do all within your power and resources to keep the "bounce" in your life, to keep an open mind about your alternatives and, finally, to age with grace. Are they, after all, so very different? On the subject of growing old, as in many of these shared moments with these remarkable women, we feel the pervasive sensation of "universality."

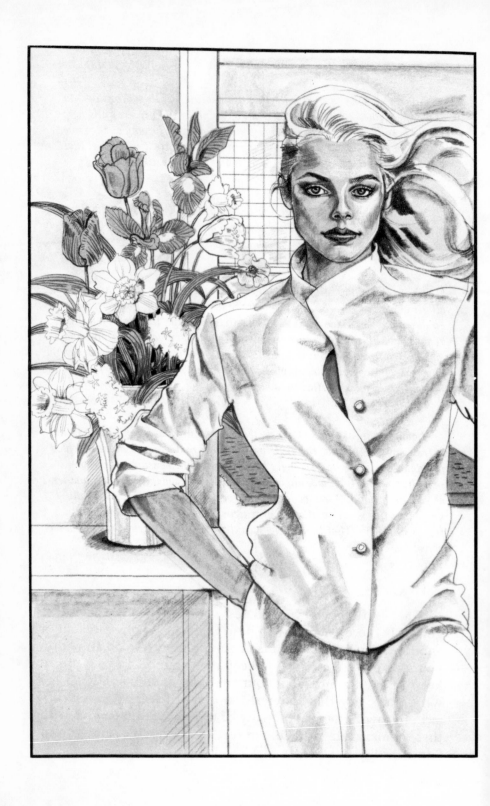

Margaux Hemingway

BEAUTY DOES NOT REST on appearance alone. I mean what really matters has to do with the inside. With your level of self-awareness. You've got to be honest with yourself and know who you are. It's instinct. You do what's right for *you* and it's fine. Tricks can't make you beautiful. The secret is having your head together."

"Do you believe, then, that anyone can be beautiful?"

"Of course!"

She's still a kid. She's five-feet-twelve ("Men may be six feet tall, but ladies are five-feet-twelve!"). She gets "into" things; she fasts, she skis like one of the guys, she's been known to take broiling-hot saunas and then jump into a tub of ice. She once weighed 180 pounds. Now she says her whole life's a diet, but she'll binge on spaghetti *and* tacos when the moon is full. She spells her name like the wine she says her parents were drinking the night she was conceived. She's got eyebrows like Groucho Marx. One of the most spectacular beauties around, her name is Margaux Hemingway; and yes, she is his granddaughter.

Margaux is the girl you'd want for a kid sister. She's a pleasure to have around, even borrowing your cashmeres. She smiles a lot—it's her favorite form of punctuation. She's easy, relaxed and open to everything. In a word, she's a joy! Margaux meets you once and never forgets you. If you bump into her at Gristede's six months down the road, you can count on her remembering your first name. And, in all probability, your birth sign.

After a little while with her, you find yourself wondering how this terrific kid from Ketchum, Idaho, has made it through her "heavy success trip" and stayed so very nice. It's quite a story. It began when Margaux decided at the age of nineteen that Sun Valley wasn't big enough to satisfy her career plans. So she abandoned her skis, her fishing pole and her hiking boots and came east to New York with nothing but herself and that name to seek her fortune.

And one night, not too long after her first time in "the Big Town," Margaux stepped through the door at a party thrown in Halston's home in honor of Liza Minnelli's anniversary and everyone—but *everyone*—turned around.

"Who *is* that fabulous girl?" Thus Margaux became The Face. She was photographed by the finest photographers, flown all over the world for fashion layouts, and blanketed the editorial sections and covers of nearly every major fashion and news magazine. Then one morning she woke up, rolled over and signed on the dotted line with Fabergé. Presto! Margaux Hemingway, the kid from Ketchum, Idaho, turned supermodel, then superbeauty, and became "The Million Dollar Babe."

It's a thrill to have a cosmetics and perfume line built around you. Margaux uses all those Babe products, too. They're all over the apartment. And, getting to know her, you can easily believe that she would take a ride in an inner tube with her man and her designer crepe de chine, scented head to toe with Babe perfume.

She's that, alright. We met in her brand-new New York apartment. Fabulous! All soft and natural (the apartment *and* "the Babe"). All the colors are gentle and neutral—nothing too razzmatazz—and all befitting her new, more quiet and introspective life-style. No more parties until dawn. She cooks, she reads, and she listens to music. "I'm more thoughtful of myself now. And, hopefully, more thoughtful of others.

"This is a place of my own, where I can go to think and read and get away from everything. All the shapes will be pure. I want everything round and soft, with clean lines. Sensuous."

Her speech is sibilant. She has a charming little lisp that sounds like the vocal on "All I Want for Christmas Is My Two Front Teeth." There is an intimacy about it that holds you in rapt attention. It's hypnotizing.

"I believe in taking quiet time, alone time. When I can schedule it, I do TM (Transcendental Meditation). That's super important to my general well-being. So are sports. Physical activity is crucial to me. The more I do, the more energy I have. I have to exercise every night. I need to run, walk, ride, fence, ski—whatever I can get into at the time. I never get tense. It probably has a lot to do with my physical activity. Tension is real bad for the face, too. That's the first place it shows. When I feel it starting, I just get up and *do* something. You know, with all those hands on you when you're being worked over for photography—one person doing your make-up, another doing your hair (and maybe doing it *all wrong* and how do you tell them without hurting their feelings because they're all tense and a little insecure), somebody buckling shoes on your feet, and they hurt—well, sometimes I get to the point where I could scream! Aaaagh! I have to shake it out. Exercise. It makes everything okay again."

There is a very definite sensuality in that voice. It's throaty and low, and somewhat leisurely. But hers is the face of the scrubbed ingenue. In a couple of years, this girl could really have power on the screen. It must be due, in part, to the relaxed way she asserts herself as a free person. She's an individual. And it has little, if anything, to do with her youth. You can believe that she just came down from a snowswept mountain.

"After I take a shower I usually stand on my head." Of course, of course. It's good for the circulation, you see.

"I'm five-feet-twelve. I've always wanted to be five-feet-sixteen, but I never made it.

"I always loved being tall. It's very sexy, being tall. You just stand up straight and no matter what you're wearing, it's sexy. I mean, with nothing showing at all."

"Okay, but what did you do at the Senior Prom, when you were taller than . . ."

"I never went to the Senior Prom."

"Oh?"

"I went to the Cowboy Prom.

"I think fasting from time to time is a beauty thing, you know? It has to do with more than weight loss. The weight loss is wonderful, but that's not all there is to fasting. I believe that you are what you eat, like Adelle Davis said. Fasting can clean out your whole body and spirit. Once I fasted for seven days. It's hard to put yourself into it at first. I mean, you really have to want to do it. But it's so good for you. My head was so high. It's very spiritual. I could feel myself rising; I became all liquid. It was beautiful!

"I have tremendous respect for the ladies of the land who are old and very together. I love the idea of growing old and getting wrinkles. It's so . . . healthy! Like my grandmother. She's full of energy. And she has a vision. Aging is a natural and healthy process.

"Perfume is one of my favorite things. I use it all the time. It's one of the things I do for the man I love and for myself. I love the smell of clean skin."

When she laughs, it comes clear from her feet. The entire length of that glorious six-foot body gets involved.

"What is your best beauty feature?"

"My eyebrows. They're also the most controversial!"

"What about your worst? Is there something you really don't like?"

"There's nothing I don't like. I've got very strong legs, for example, and they could be a problem if I thought about it but I don't mind them because they're a part of me and my heritage. They're my father's and his father's legs. They're great for sports. I look like my father's side of the family, like my grandfather, and I'm proud."

She's as spirited as a filly. Her joy is contagious. Everything about Margaux makes you wish you were young again and living the special life she leads. She's a Cinderella who could care less about the ball, the glass slipper and the chichi rigmarole.

Shown a 105.54-carat diamond called the Soleil d'Or (golden sun) during a taping of a French talk show she commented that, yes, big girls need big diamonds. ("But that one was so big it looked fake.") Then she tossed it up in the air and caught it in her teeth. "I'm real good at peanuts, too!" she added.

"Okay, I believe that beauty comes from within, first of all. Ugly people don't bother me, because no one is really ugly. It's the personality of the person I look for. And with some people, there's this very special something. Their beauty comes shining out through them, they have a *light* within them as clear and bright as a star. Those people are the really beautiful people, the ones with that shining inner light. That's what I would like to have, more than fame, more than money, more than anything else."

And you do, Margaux. Yes, you do.

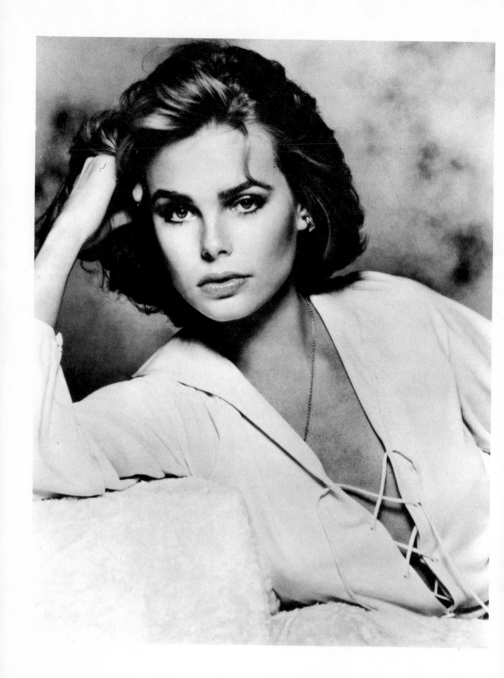

"I think you can be ugly and still be beautiful. What really matters has to do with the inside. You've got to be honest with yourself and know who you are."

MAKEUP:
Margaux Hemingway

"DOING YOUR FACE is like painting a portrait. I'm an artist and when I do careful makeup I like to structure my face the same way I would model an object on the canvas. Makeup can be an art form. But most of the time, I just don't bother!"

Margaux Hemingway the fabulous *Babe* looks absolutely terrific with a clean face. She chooses to stay as natural-looking as possible because, she says, frankly it's easier that way. She spends her time in other ways. But when she goes the whole route, she follows the expert makeup advice and technique of Way Bandy, the most fashionable and famous face-maker of them all. Way taught her all about her beauty, back when she first came to work in New York at nineteen. That, she confesses, is *really* the way to learn. From the best expert in the business.

When she has a heavy business day coming up or is to be photographed she does the following: First a light coat of moisturizer. Over that she applies a sheer, pale foundation. When it has set a little she adds a second layer, this time in a shade that is a bit darker than the first. Her cheek color is generally a powder and she applies it with one of her vast and varied collection of Japanese art brushes which, she says, are

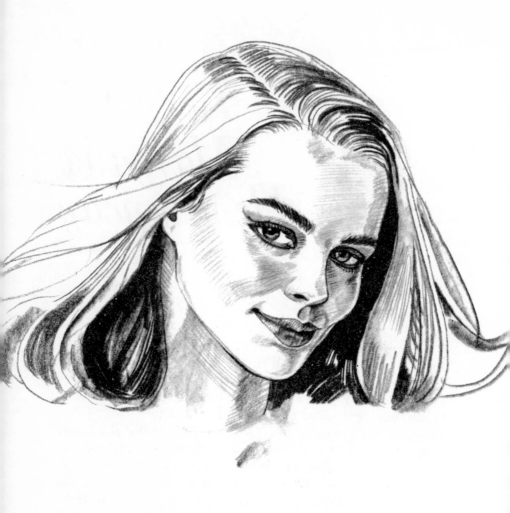

MARGAUX HEMINGWAY

THE BASE: *Moisturizer; light, sheer foundation; then another coat of foundation, slightly darker than the first. Powder blusher. Baby powder to set.*

THE EYES: *Either shadow or mascara. Shadow soft and neutral.*

THE MOUTH: *Natural lip liner pencil. Clear gloss.*

THE FINISHED LOOK: *Healthy, glowing. Her youthful face and clear skin do all the talking!*

available at art supply stores or in Japanese variety shops. The sealer is a light dusting of baby powder. *Baby powder!* Straight from the plastic Johnson & Johnson container. She loves baby products, finds them gentle and hygienic and she enjoys the clean fragrance. The cosmetic line she prefers, of course, is the Babe collection from Fabergé.

Her famous feature is the fantastic heavy brows. Having such strong eyebrows causes her to be careful about her eye makeup. Too little and your eyes disappear. Too much and the rest of your face drops right off the map. Surprisingly, Margaux rarely uses both shadow and mascara. She chooses one or the other. Her eyes are a beautiful blue-grey. She told us she'd *love* to be able to wear contacts. Then she would put an orange contact on the left and purple on the right. (That *is* what she said.) Like a space lady. And then she'd coordinate them with a bathing suit. (Sometimes Margaux can get a little bizarre.) But she laughed after that statement, so we assume she was joking.

Margaux's mouth is full and extremely sensual. She rarely uses a strong lip color (especially since filming *Lipstick*, she added), preferring a natural lip pencil and clear gloss.

A complete makeup job takes her between thirty and forty-five minutes. But this is not her everyday timetable. She's not really into makeup per se. She doesn't collect lipsticks or experiment with colored shadows. In fact, she seems to have a hard time holding on to her favorite lip liner pencil. "Things are always floating around in here. I lose everything. I never seem to have a bobby pin or a rubber band. I guess makeup is not the area of my greatest attention."

Margaux also told us she once plucked those landmark brows of hers. Then she went out to play a rousing game of tennis. It was a major turning point in her beauty life. Why? The sweat came pouring down over those new, delicate eyebrows and into the no-nonsense blue eyes below and she couldn't see the ball. She lost the match. "That's what eyebrows are there for. To keep the sweat out of your eyes! I'll never pluck them again."

$\mathscr{L}ove$

LOVE. They all had a lot to say about it. It's no wonder. When you look as good as they do, we imagine the subject must come up pretty often. And in interesting ways. How many proposals of marriage do you suppose Cheryl Ladd receives by mail in one week? And she's a married lady! Consider the sweet nothings whispered in Suzanne Somers' little pink ear by her stage door Johnnies. ("Yesterday I walked out of CBS after a taping without any makeup on or anything, and there were hundreds of people and all these strange men waiting for me. Most of them had cameras.") How much of an asset (and how much of a liability) is being a public beauty in matters of the heart? As a society, we tend to equate being beautiful with being deserving of love. Imagine, then, the situation among the crème de la crème, the *very* beautiful. Do they have to ask themselves, "Does he love me for myself or for my beauty?" You say you'd like to have that problem? We wonder. After the last adulatory adjective is written about each of them, we wonder if we'd ever want to trade places. At least the average woman knows it's her self and not the envy of millions of other men he's after. When you look like Jacqueline Bisset, whom can you trust?

Before we get a word deeper into this chapter, we have to tell you that their relationships seemed confusing at times. Someone we interviewed in her cozy little cottage for two on Thursday was freelancing again by Sunday afternoon. At one point we got to thinking that we were involved in some strange way. No sooner would we transcribe the interview than ppfffft! End of the marriage. Was all of this connected with their being beautiful? Clearly they live by a different set of rules and an unusual assortment of dos and don'ts. But, surprisingly, most of them had some pretty conventional attitudes about love and marriage and children—as well as about jealousy. We guess, when you get down to it, even though their fights make headlines on the front pages of the *Star* and the *Enquirer*, they aren't all that different from the rest of the romantic world. Their romances might be blown out of proportion, but their love dreams are still recognizable.

Take the question of careers. All of them who commented on the subject said that a successful relationship had to be built around an understanding of the problems of forced separation. Each of the married ones said she firmly believed she and her husband had solved those problems. On Thursday, that is. Or whatever day we happened to interview them. But it's a cold, hard fact that it's nearly impossible to keep a marriage on the track when you have to make reservations months in advance to see your husband or wife between jobs. Those of us who are working wives know the problems. Romance can fly out the window when Saturday night is the only available time to do the wash. Imagine how it must be when distance is added to schedule. Or when he's working dawn to dusk and she's idle and bored. Without, of course, so much as the wash to do because her traditional home-type duties have been taken care of by somebody else. And, of course, there is the constant presence of available men (or women) who think your spouse is 1) divine, and/or 2) a romantic one-way ticket to overnight success. Groupies aren't a factor for most of us. They are here.

So we deal in this chapter with the subject of love among the beautiful with a modicum of irreverence and a great deal of sympathy for the inhabitants of this world turned upside down. For the ladies who would love to be loved for their poetry, or their intellect, or their craft or, quite simply, for themselves—as well as for their beauty.

Now, seriously, would you trade places?

You might with Mary Tyler Moore. Mary's been married (sounds like a song title) for sixteen years to Grant Tinker. Not only are they a long-run husband and wife, they are each other's best friend. Her descriptions of their quiet private evenings at home, sharing dinner and shop talk in front of the fire, are positively Rodgers and Hart. When one or the other must travel alone, they miss each other terribly. So much so that, to make up for the separations, they vacation as a twosome at least once a year. Hawaii is such a favorite romantic retreat, Mary keeps a special wardrobe for Hawaiian escapes. Grant's personal likes and dislikes play a big part in Mary's decisions—right down to and including her nail color (although, as you know, she usually opts for color rather than his choice of natural nails). And Grant is just as involved as Mary in her professional decisions—so involved, in fact, she says she couldn't imagine life without him, or with any other man. Could this stability and ongoing love be the prime reason that she fairly bursts with confidence and security? Mary is a model of loving commitment. She doesn't even indulge in harmless flirtation. She's not antiflirting—in fact, she thinks it's a "terrific sport!"—but feels that it's best left to the woman (or man) who's looking. And who's looking? Not Mary. In fact, she's not too happy when other women even *look* at Grant.

"I'm potentially a very jealous woman! I guess it's a sign of my respect for his attractiveness. But I never feel as if I'm in competition for his love, or that I have to stay on my toes to keep it. If I were sick and looked terrible, I would never say, 'I don't want him to see me like this.' When I'm down with the flu and look like something the cat dragged in, my first thought is still, 'Where's my husband!' I want him with me, no matter what. And Grant is always there when I need him."

Another woman with a remarkably stable marriage is Ann-

Margret. She and Roger Smith have been married for twelve years now. Ann-Margret is very proud of that. Her successful relationship with her husband gives her as much a feeling of accomplishment as those two Oscar nominations. She works at her marriage just as hard as she works at her career. No marriage, she says, is a success on its own. You've got to be willing to devote time and effort to make it work. Particularly when you're in a profession where you're filming in one town or another this week and doing a nightclub act in Vegas the next. In the end, it wasn't what she said about her love for him that impressed us as much as the extent to which he influences her life. Roger is her master builder. He created that incredible closet and dressing room. He designed her special swingout hairdryer. And, most important, he's in on all of her career decisions from A to Z. Roger is clearly the center of her universe and, as such, he gives her strength and self-confidence. It was waking up four days after the famous Tahoe fall and seeing him sitting at her bedside that convinced her that she was going to pull through. In short, we have the distinct impression that it is he who packages her, wraps her up and ties the bow for all the world to see. And she, in turn, gives him all the love she can muster. And coming from Ann-Margret, that's a whole lot of love.

Ask Suzanne Somers about her love life and she'll tell an incredible story. It seems that the first time she laid eyes on Alan she fell head over heels in love. And that, friends, was ten years ago. A few years ago they were married. Why the wait? Suzanne says they had some pretty basic differences of opinion on several major issues. Like conflicting careers. On the very day they solved the last of them to their mutual satisfaction, they filed for the license.

Suzanne is, to say the least, a realist when it comes to marriage.

"Alan is ten years older than I and he had some very definite ideas about the man being the dominant one, being the *boss*. I never burned my bra or anything like that, but I do believe in equality. I don't buy the idea of 'bosses,' not even from the man I love. I was crazy about him all those years, there never was anyone else for me, but a marriage then just wouldn't have worked. I had had my one disaster. I wasn't about to have a second!"

So, Suzanne, how is the marriage working, two years down that rocky road? She gives it a ten—A-one letter perfect. "Loving Alan, knowing that he loves me, has a lot to do with how I feel about myself, and about my self-confidence. A lot of men come on to me now, because of the show and all the publicity. Total strangers, some of them. And men who wouldn't have given me the time of day three years ago. All that attention can be a difficult thing to handle. But I'm not even tempted. Not a one of them can hold a candle to Alan. I just can't take my eyes off my husband!"

But is she confident about his love for her? Sure! Of course! Well, maybe. Suzanne, the realist, says you never can be sure who's lurking around that next corner. "When another woman turns her headlights on Alan, it can really drive me mad. It's amazing how threatened I feel. I guess all of us, no matter how secure we think we are, are vulnerable and can be very badly hurt. I know that he loves me, but I can't control my emotional reaction at the thought of losing him."

Cheryl Ladd says flat out that finding the right man and sticking with him is the basis for everything else in life. That kind of love, that solidarity, helps you to get in touch with yourself and your belief in your talent and your abilities. It's the core. And the sure test is that you have to really like yourself with the man. If he makes you feel good about yourself, he's the one. Then, when you realize that you're terrific, you no longer need to feel jealous of anyone else. Cheryl *hates* jealousy. She finds it totally paralyzing. No one who is constantly wishing to be someone else can ever get anywhere in life.

Cheryl is one woman who seems to have it all together— her self-image, her marriage, her family and her career. She's got balance. You can tell. And David (who is Alan Ladd's son and has been Cheryl's husband for five years now) seems to be comfortable with Cheryl and the dramatic upswing in her career. Then there's little Jordan, age three, whom they both adore. Well, here's hoping . . .

The next group weren't quite so successful. When we first talked with Margaux Hemingway, she was a brand-new bride, full of plans and promises and decorating ideas. The marriage crashed. We certainly hope she did better in the drapery department. She's since moved on to her second and, it would appear, more long-lasting marriage. Back then, she did say the one thing she never was and never could be is a flirt. She talks to men on a buddy-to-buddy basis. She hates it—simply hates it—when women use their femininity (or their sensuality) to get their way, either personally or professionally. So it's probably safe to assume that that first marriage didn't go thud because Margaux batted her "Oh, you Babe" blue eyes at anyone else. And since she also said she was immune to jealousy (due, she claimed, to a strong level of self-respect and self-confidence) we've got to eliminate the green-eyed monster. Who knows in these matters? And since she's moved along quite happily to husband #2, it's hardly worth discussing.

Marisa Berenson, on the other hand, was another story. Somehow the consequences of this mobile life-style with its storybook ups and dramatic downs seem more poignant when you remember the children. Sitting with Marisa, watching her fondle her tiny new baby, then hearing several days later that she and Jim Randall had separated, really affected us. Had we sensed a sort of detachment, a strangeness, that afternoon? She seemed very tired, but then, who isn't, even with household help, with a newborn? It makes the fantasy of that house more mysterious knowing that she vanished with her child so soon after we visited it. She had said so little about her life with her husband, had barely responded to our questions about the role love played in her life. She did have this to say about jealousy:

"I am a very feminine person. I love to have people, including men, notice me when I enter a room. But when that happens to my husband, when other women notice him, rather than upsetting me, it pleases me. I enjoy knowing that my husband is attractive to other women. I would hate to have a husband no one would look at! I can only imagine myself getting jealous or upset out of extreme personal hurt. And then, well, I have my belief that things happen for the best."

She must have known what was about to happen in her life. Was she reconciled even then?

Then there was Phyllis. Phyllis George Evans. Well at least she *was* when we first talked to her. For about four months. Now, even moving in this set, four-month marriages are unusual. We interviewed Phyllis twice: once in New York, pre-romance; and again in L.A., several months later and after the nuptials. At the time we felt it was necessary to update her feelings and style to fit her new California-married-lady situation. We should have waited a few weeks.

This is not to say that things didn't look swell at the time. The Evans' domicile did look a tad like a bachelor pad—full of strong, man-sized furniture covered in leathers and dark brown velvets—but we got the distinct impression that Phyllis had pastel plans. The bridegroom did take the time to come in to meet us, kiss his new bride, and assure her he would be breaking up his prolonged business meeting shortly so that they could manage to lunch together by three (she looked awfully hungry). It was terribly friendly, cordial and connubial.

Phyllis had some amusing comments on the subject of marriage and career that afternoon. Take the story of her adjustment to Bob's checkup phone calls. Seems he had a habit of ringing the house on a whim between his multimillion-dollar dealings at Paramount, just to say "Howdy!" If Phyllis happened to be out shopping or having her nails done (you should be smiling at this!), he would become concerned about her whereabouts and start leaving "Call me" messages all over town. When she returned his call(s) later in the day, the opening line would be something like, "Where have you been!", followed by "I've been calling you all day and you haven't been at home" and sealed with a "Why didn't you call me, darling?". (The "darling" should make it all better, you see!) But Phyllis had been independent too long to be comfortable in that love-yoke.

One advantage of her busy professional schedule and constant traveling was that it got her away for a few days and made her returns very exciting. "It's just like a honeymoon when I come home!" she told us. Well, maybe not *exactly* like a honeymoon, but better than being around day after day, having to be constantly pulled together and anticipating visitors, living in an industry "open house" with big business being juggled in the pool cabanas, the screening room, on the tennis courts and along the private jogging trails. Phyl told us that on that very morning, her mother called her from Texas with news of an unexpected tidbit in the gossip columns of a national weekly. It read:

"PHYLLIS GEORGE HAS ALREADY LEFT BOB EVANS' BED FOR ANOTHER!"

"Oh, yeh!" laughed Phyl. "That was the week before last when I was covering tobogganing in Canada. The other bed was at the Statler Hilton."

We left for New York. But the gossip didn't die down. And soon after the word was out. How was it they put it?

"We're still good friends," says Phyllis George about her split from hubby, Bob Evans, "but our careers tore our marriage apart."

Glib, isn't it? That sort of announcement fairly reeks of easy come, easy go when it appears on the pages of *Silver Screen* or the like. Don't be misled by the tone of those press releases. Divorce among the beautiful is no less painful than it is for the rest of us. And being beautiful doesn't make being alone any easier. In truth, it probably makes being alone more frequent. In our pre-Bob interview, riding down to the lobby from her thirtieth-floor apartment, Phyllis confided, "You know, I spend a whole lot of Saturday nights alone. I guess it's part of the price you pay. Who wants to go out on agent-arranged date/appearances? Not me, for sure! And it's hard for me to get to know anyone on my own. I have a crazy work schedule to contend with and I can't just bump into a man on the street. You think you've got problems editing out the strange ones. You can't possibly imagine! I guess I'm like any other single person—full of insecurities about falling in love—and scared to death that I'll be all alone, counting off the minutes on New Year's Eve."

Isolated. Protected. Running too hard to keep up professionally. Missing a lot of the options most of us take for granted. So the next time you walk into your corner delicatessen and spot a terrific-looking guy buying sandwiches for one, and he spots you, think of Phyllis. You may go home with the guy. She goes home with the sandwich.

We're going to stop with the sad tales right here. All we can do is hope that by the time you are reading this chapter, the list won't have grown by another name. What do you think? Are we being too optimistic?

Now for a divorced but happy ending. Diane Von Furstenberg is one of the more famous single women around. She had the sort of marriage you don't walk away from easily. First off, there were the two children. Then there was the fact that she was a princess, but only because she was married to a prince. A lot of people weren't surprised. There were, after all, more rumors about that marriage than about its termination. Diane was even quoted as saying "The only way for a relationship to survive is without sex." That quotation gets more exposure than Diane's collections. We quote it again for one pertinent reason. She's changed her mind. Diane is now very much the romantic about such things as loving and being loved. Now she believes in strong relationships. In fact, she claims that she might even consider having another child. But she will not, she says, have another husband.

"I cannot live without a man. But I could never live *for* a man. Love is wonderful, but marriage is more for the men today than for the women. Men need marriage to complete their lives. Women are so liberated that they can survive very well without—can develop a good, healthy sense of themselves as complete persons and become successful—without men."

Who is she describing there? You're right. Diane. Diane is an extravagantly attractive and enormously female woman, but she talks about herself and her life post-Prince as if she herself were a man. This is the new Romantic Woman. Not wasting away for want of her lost love. When Diane feels an attack of the blues coming on, she says she takes a lover. Not for life, you understand, but for the afternoon. She carries the responsibilities and has all the independence of a man. But she has one big complaint about her brand of role reversal.

"I am the head of my family. Everyone depends upon me. I run a multimillion-dollar business. But the terrible thing is that I have no one at home to care for my household and my personal day-to-day business. What I need is a wife."

The Seventies has heard this line before.

Jackie Bisset's relationship with Vic Dray keeps getting better. This is due in part, according to Jackie, to the fact that Vic is becoming more and more successful professionally. There's something intrinsically sexy about a successful man, says Jackie. There's got to be a lot of truth in that. In fact he's *got* to be successful if he's involved with an enormously successful woman. Everyone agreed on this point. Most love relationships self-destruct if her career is going like gangbusters and his stays on ground zero. Or, worse yet, his shooting star crashes and burns. Jackie, for one, strongly advises equality. It's a requirement in her personal life. But not equality within the same business, please. At least, not if it encourages him to offer helpful advice. Jackie admits that she *craves* romance but takes great care that it doesn't get mixed up with being taken care of financially. For her love is pure, unadulterated pleasure. She is, by far, the most sensual woman we met. Spontaneously sensual. Jackie can walk into a room and fall wildly in love with a stranger in the crowd, even if she will never see him again. And love is a very honest business with her. She is looking for neither husband nor children. She says she's too smart for that. All around her, marriages are tumbling down—there's just no continuity in Hollywood. Even though she tends to one-man-one-woman relationships, she firmly believes that no love, no matter how overwhelming it may seem, is forever.

"You ask me about love. Well, I'll tell you that I have a very realistic attitude toward love and marriage. I don't accept the condition of monogamy. 'Forever' is an intolerably long time. Love can happen many times in a lifetime. It's never the same. Like people, it's constantly changing, growing or receding, a living thing rather than a static condition. I seriously doubt that I will ever marry, although when I am in love, I can never imagine being with another man. Being in love, being with a man I love, is an essential part of my being alive."

When she is in love, Jackie says her appearance suffers. It's tough to be up all night and look divine the next morning. Circles under the eyes and a smile on the lips are a sure sign! After the first few days, she tends to look a bit bleary-eyed and her edges get frayed. This is due not only to the hours she keeps, but to her devotion to her lover—to the exclusion of self-indulgent things like makeup or meals. Under those circumstances, she practically has to leave town to get herself back together. When she is away on business and has nothing to occupy her after-hours, she'll fuss and primp and, in general, get herself prepared for a glorious homecoming—just so she can let it all fall apart again, deliciously, with her lover. Love is so central in her life, she has to watch herself to keep it all in balance. There is a conflict in her between giving herself over to the joy of loving another and the strong sense of separateness so necessary to her individual personality and her work. She is a battleground between sense and sensuality.

Love among the superbeauties. The intensity of their need to be loved should surprise none of us. After all, they are loved publicly, each of them. It's not hard to accept their need to be loved on a more private personal level as well. But it is fascinating how many of them admitted to difficulties in finding a fulfilling love relationship because of their high visibility and their isolation. We could hardly believe how few really found *themselves* beautiful. "Why are you including me in this? I'm really not beautiful, you know. I'm very flattered that you want to talk with me at all." We heard it over and over again. The same need to be reassured of this most obvious fact. The same desire to be cared for by the men in their lives (not to be confused with "taken care of"). The need to be needed as *women*. To be comforted ("Whenever I'm ill, all I want is my husband"), to be loved purely and simply for themselves. "Tell me, if I were to grow old tomorrow—if I were no longer beautiful—would you still love me just the same?" These are universal needs. They are understandable to every one of us and they come from the mouths of these glorious women who we imagined had no fears—no insecurities about their beauty or being deserving of love.

Liv Ullmann, in her sensitive, straightforward way, responded, "There is no such thing as beauty alone and to itself. Beauty, real beauty, exists only between people. I am beautiful because I reflect the beauty radiating from another person. We are two mirrors, held up one to the other. Love is the primary requirement, not the shape of the mouth, the color of the eyes, the clarity of the skin. Love. Loving and being loved. Then anyone who makes you feel beautiful by loving you as a friend or as a lover becomes a beautiful person in your eyes because he has touched something in you that needed to be touched. Life is relentless, demanding and, often, terribly disappointing. But if you are in love, that is all that matters. That is all the beauty in the world."

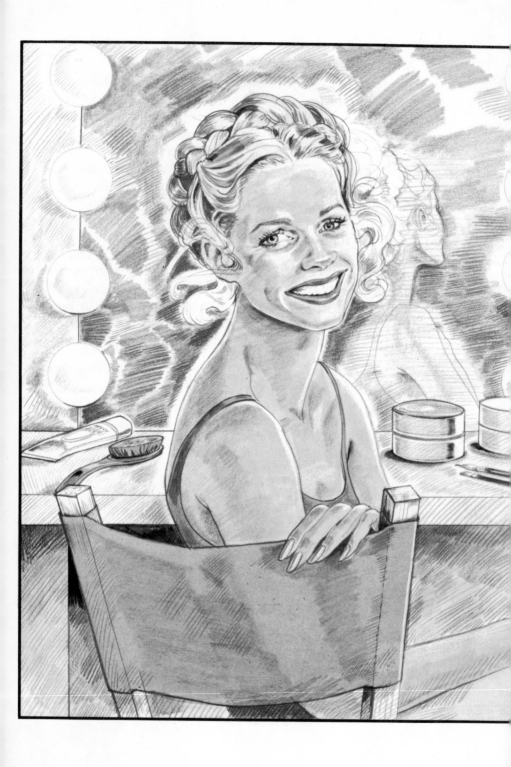

Liv Ullmann

"I FEEL THAT beauty is of two kinds. One is outward superficial beauty, if you happen to havè a beautiful face or are clever at doing makeup. The other is the beauty of the interior, that comes from within. I have found that the easier one, if you are aware of it and work to let it show, is the beauty from within. If you feel good about yourself and it is a sunny day inside, the sun will shine through you and make you beautiful."

Liv Ullmann sits on a folding chair, her long legs drawn up under her Indian-style, in the dusty and abused star dressing room of the Imperial Theater. Even though there are photographs scattered around of her child, her friends, herself, and a few fresh pillows on the faded chintz sofa, it has the look of a rented room. There is nothing glamorous about it. Except Liv Ullmann. Liv isn't glamorous in the usual way. There is nothing chic or flashy about her. Quite simply she has presence. Here is a glamour of natural style, of human warmth, of reputation and of consummate professional skill. When you look at her, you see far more than a pleasant woman. All that she can do with that expressive face and body is written in her eyes.

She is sitting there in that unladylike position, her cheeks flushed from the baseball game she's abandoned to come and talk with us. Her very female body is folded up. She wears a black leotard, a peasant skirt and no makeup at all. Her kindness comes through the famous throaty voice.

"The outward beauty can sometimes make others feel uncomfortable. That is unfortunate. So I concern myself with the inner beauty only. I feel that is the best because it makes others feel good about themselves. It doesn't threaten."

She is here in New York to star in the revival of Eugene O'Neill's *Anna Christie,* which she has interpreted to be a play about liberation. Her portrayal of the highly three-dimensional character of Anna has drawn both applause and very favorable reviews and the Imperial is filled night after night. It's difficult to imagine the lights and applause back here in this cubbyhole.

It was our first time backstage in a New York theater. The watchman at the stage door smelled of cigars and wasn't friendly. (In all those Dick Powell–Ruby Keeler movies, he was "Pop" and everybody loved him. Where is *that* character and who is *this* man?) The walls are covered with graffiti, names and numbers and assorted brief résumés. This landmark, this mausoleum, was built in 1925. The labyrinthian back halls show their age. The Imperial is an aging female lead, full of fond memories. *Rose-Marie* played here. And Gertrude Lawrence became a star on this stage in *Oh, Kay!* written by George and Ira Gershwin in 1926. Then there was *Call Me Madam!* with Ethel Merman in 1950, *Carnival* in 1961, and the longest-running musical ever in the long history of Broadway—*Fiddler on the Roof* in 1968. Back here there is dust. Out in front, magic.

"I am interested in people. It shows in everything I do, in the way I approach them, in the way I act. I listen to them. I am interested in what they say and I am generous with myself. When you approach people in this way a kind of beauty comes from you to them and it is reflected in them and they return it to you. I have benefited from this beauty in relationships because I am not a beautiful woman. I am not good with makeup or with putting dresses together. I am happy with myself and with others. I am enthusiastic about people and that is my strength."

Her speaking voice is rich and full and sensual; the slight lilt of her accent and a few awkward English phrases add to its immense charm. She overflows with a *kind* sensuality and she talks freely about its effect on the people around her, particularly the men.

"I suppose I have a special way of relating to the men I find attractive. A good friend of mine, a man who has known me for a long time, says, 'You look at them in that special way that says "take care of me and my feelings."' If someone calls me the next day, my friend will laugh and say to me 'Liv! You *looked* at him!' It must be true that I communicate something that appeals. We have all noticed how people, especially men, will sometimes single out a particular woman who we might find ordinary and yet she will capture his attention. I think people look for more than beauty in a woman. It is a sort of radiance. The feeling of 'I'd like to know you. I like you. Who are you and what do you feel?' A woman who is concerned with her superficial physical beauty, you see, has a hard time communicating this message to others. She is too busy with her appearance."

The phone is ringing. A secretary in blue jeans snatches it up and starts chatting pleasantly. It distracts us for a second. A masseur is waiting in the hall. There's a discrete knock on the door to announce him. Still, she is a center of calm. In less than an hour she will become Anna, the disenchanted daughter turned whore turned wife. It is a difficult and demanding role. But there is no feeling of tension or hurry on her face. The pale eyes are attentive to us and her full soft mouth is settled in a reflective half-smile. Behind her on the dressing table we can see flowers in a vase. Not roses. Field flowers.

"Personal attractiveness is sometimes a safety device. I think this is necessary, particularly in business. You known the feeling: I am prepared. I am combed and manicured and my clothes are just right and my face is just right. I am safe. I can be looked at closely and remain secure about myself. I don't know whether I feel more beautiful then, but the fences are up and I feel protected and safe. This can be crucial in business. But in your personal life, I think it is a little better when all the fences are down, when you are a little more vulnerable." (She pronounces it "voolnerable" and turns it into a new word with new depth and meaning.) "When you are more vulnerable you are more human. There is a special kind of beauty that comes from vulnerability."

Yes, she is that. It is, in part, what her friend says she communicates to men. But it goes much farther. She has written about her feelings, discussed her womanliness and her loves openly in her book. She makes no secret of having lived by impulse and been guided by emotion. *Changing* is both realistic and romantic, as is the woman who wrote it.

"I have a realistic attitude about myself. I am not a beauty. I have no beautiful features. I do not use makeup because only women with beautiful features should use makeup. The rest of us look better without. When I went to Hollywood to film *Lost Horizon* and *Forty Carats,* they tried. Oh, how hard they tried to make me beautiful. They shaded and powdered and glossed, but in the end I just looked awful. Not at all like myself. That is why I use nothing on the stage. A little mascara and lip gloss, but nothing else. Then, when I blush, I *blush* and it is real blood that rises up in my cheeks and not the creams. My skin is receptive to the color of the lights. My hair is natural too. I prefer it long and free like this. Then I can use it as I use any part of my body when I act or am with people. In Hollywood they told me if I would just let them cut and style my hair they could make me a movie star. I said no. No, you may not touch my hair. It is part of me this way and it stays."

Liv is not a young girl. We know that. Her child is approaching adolescence. But she has a youthfulness that makes it impossible to pinpoint her age. And with her, it really doesn't matter.

"There is a young girl in me who refuses to grow up," she says. "Having a child has made me aware of how far away I have come from my own childhood. I can relive it with my daughter, but at the same time I see it from a distance, from another place. I can watch it but I can never live it again. There are many things in life, and in love, like this. Bittersweet. A child can redirect your center of interest away from yourself, which is a wonderful kind of love. But it is also the kind of love that teaches to love when you sometimes get nothing in return. It is pleasurable and painful, both. These things, I think, help us to develop our femininity."

She talks comfortably about love and loving. Lynn is her child by Ingmar Bergman. Their private/working relationship was and is complex and fascinating. She is clearly one of the few women who could first work with a man, then live with him and have his child, and then separate but continue to work together, year after year, long after the romance has gone. She speaks of him with warm affection. There is no bitterness. He is still very much a part of her life and career.

"Doing what you *love* to do in life, loving whom you choose to love, this is happiness and the best beauty asset. Living your dreams. Being able to fulfill your talent and your wishes. Whatever it is that really is you makes all the difference. You are then secure with yourself. You are beautiful. Long ago, when I was engaged to my husband, I was the ugly duckling. My best friend met me then with my fiancé and she and her husband were horrified by me. 'What can we do to help him get rid of that girl?' they said to each other. But living out my fantasies and my dreams has taken me far from that plain, awkward young girl I was. Working toward what I wanted for myself professionally, and finding love wherever it was, have allowed me to grow into the woman I am."

There are more insistent rappings on the door. We gather up our papers and leave Liv to her massage and preparations. But we don't want it to end there in that dismal little hallway with handshakes and quick goodbyes. So we go to the box office and buy a pair of the last seats for this next-to-closing performance in the grand old Imperial Theater. We sit, way off to one side, barely able to see the stage and wait to meet Anna.

Midway through the first act, she enters for the first time. . . .

(ANNA CHRISTOPHERSON enters. She is a tall, blond, fully-developed girl of twenty, handsome after a large, Viking-daughter fashion, but now run down in health and plainly showing all of the outward evidences of belonging to the world's oldest profession. Her youthful face is already hard and cynical beneath its layer of makeup. Her clothes are the tawdry finery of peasant stock turned prostitute. She comes and sinks wearily in a chair by the table left front.)

ANNA: Gimme a whisky—ginger ale on the side. And don't be stingy, baby.

(That voice! Raspy, harsh, with a cutting edge of disgust and fatigue. Where did she find that voice?)

LARRY: (Sarcastically) Shall I serve it in a pail?

ANNA: (With a hard laugh) That suits me down to the ground.

She is old. She moves with heaviness and fatigue, her tall, lithe body all bent and low to the floor. This is impossible! This is not the same woman. The face is different, almost un-recognizable under that little hat and veil. We are unable to see either her hair or her eyes. Within those few minutes be-tween our leaving her there in that hallway and her entrance, she has transformed herself. Anna dominates the stage, mov-ing the others around with small gestures and her sharp tongue. She is in complete control of the role. In fact, she is in command of the entire performance.

End of Act One. Intermission. We share our enthusiasm over orange drinks. It's the first time we've seen her live like this. How different she is from her films. There's such an im-mediacy about the theater, about her acting. And to have been so close to her a few hours before, so comfortable, and then to see her up there—in character—what an experience it is!

We are unfamiliar with the play. We are not prepared for Act Two. We expect the same woman, the daughter/prostitute with her battered hat and hidden eyes.

ACT II

(SCENE: Ten days later. The stern of the deeply-laden barge, SIMEON WINTHROP, at anchor in the outer harbor of Provincetown, Mass.

(It is ten o'clock at night. Dense fog shrouds the barge on all sides, and she floats motionless on a calm.

(As the curtain rises, Anna is discovered standing near the coil of rope on which the lantern is placed. She looks healthy, transformed. The natural color has come back to her face. She has on a black oilskin coat, but wears no hat. She is staring out into the fog astern with an expression of awed wonder.)

At the sight of her, tall and straight, her yellow hair long and free around her luminous face, the audience applauds. They are so moved by the ease with which she has gone from Anna, stooped and ill, to this majestic young woman, staring off into the fog, that, spontaneously, they applaud. She was absolutely right about herself. Her skin flushes and glows under the lights. Her hair is an extension of the new, free Anna she portrays. The whole being of this character is washed clean and fresh and she has done it without words or gestures or even makeup. Her majesty, like her beauty, comes from inside.

One hour later, the curtain falls and the curtain calls begin. The applause is steady and strong as, one by one, the actors come up to the apron of the stage and take their bows.

Then Liv Ullmann steps out and the house comes down. One person here, one there, then in groups of four and five, the audience rises to its feet and the cacophony of applause fills the old Imperial. What a happy sound! She stands in the bright light of the footlights, her hair shining and wild and

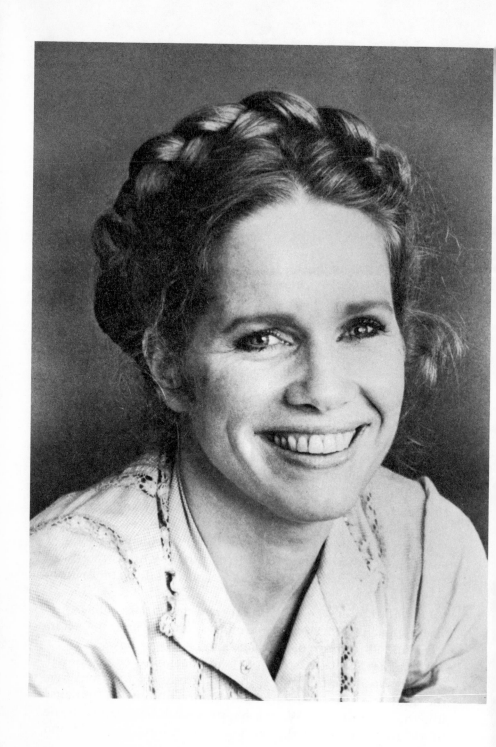

free, her lush mouth smiling in simple and grateful accep-
tance.

"And when you can communicate the beauty you feel within you to others, and it is returned to you from them, that is
the best life can be."

She is blushing. And we know it's real.

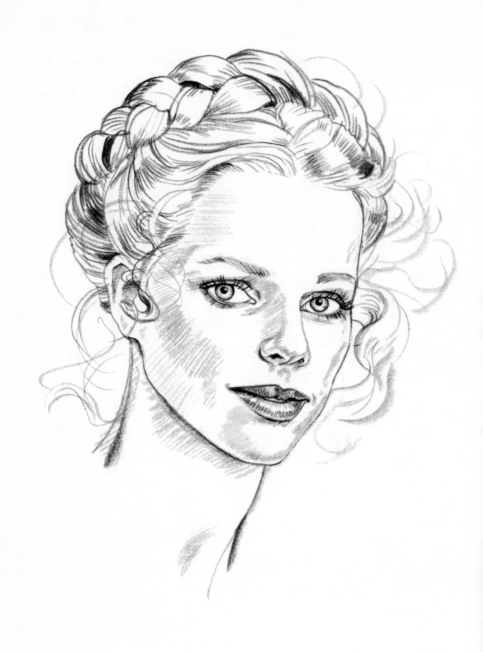

MAKEUP:

Liv Ullmann

Liv Ullmann wears no makeup at all!
She is free to show her face as is . . . and with good reason.
For Liv Ullmann, her ideal state is to be natural.